FIRST AID GUIDE

Dr. Rajeev Sharma
M.D., D.Lit

DIAMOND BOOKS

Published by : Diamond Pocket Books (P) Ltd.
X-30, Okhla Industrial Area, Phase-II
New Delhi-110 020
Phone : 011-40712200
E-mail : sales@dpb.in
Website : www.dpb.in
Printed by : Repro (India)

FIRST AID GUIDE (*An Exhaustive Guide for All those who Value Life!*
By : Dr. Rajeev Sharma

Preface

In most situations that require first aid, there will be no life-threatening danger. You will simply be assisting a conscious casualty; whose recovery from some minor injury or illness is not in doubt. In all cases, your aim is to work to a plan and discover what is wrong with the casualty, and to give prompt, correct treatment in a methodical way.

Before tending to a casualty, however, you must survey the whole scene. Your first responsibility is to make sure that the area is safe. Often hazards such as passing traffic can be dealt with simply, but where the danger is too great or too imminent, you may need to move the casualty even at the risk of aggravating the injury. Do this only if it is safe to approach the casualty: you cannot help others if you also become a casualty. Only when the casualty is safe you can begin to treat the illness or injury.

The First Aider Should:

- Preserve life
- Pay strict attention to safety
- Follow the ABC of resuscitation
- Control any major bleeding
- Limit worsening of the condition
- Make a diagnosis of the injury or illness, if possible, by means of a thorough examination.
- Give priority to seriously injured casualties.
- Treat multiple injuries in order of priority dealing with life-

threatening conditions first. Consider the possibility of hidden secondary conditions.

- Promote the casualty's recovery.
- Relieve any discomfort, pain or anxiety. Arrange for appropriate medical attention.

All these aspects and the major problems where first aid is required has been discussed in this book for the benefit of the readers.

Dr. Rajeev Sharma
email : drs108@gmail.com

A brief about Dr. Rajeev Sharma

Dr. Rajeev Sharma is an eminent consultant of Homoeopathy,Yoga, Naturopathy and Alternative Medicine in India. He has written more than two hundred twenty five books (225) in Hindi and English and around one thousand articles which have been published in various newspapers and magazines. He is also an Editional Board Member of the prestigious *Asian Homoeopathic Journal* besides many other newspapers and magazines.

Dr. Rajeev Sharma has written books on ayurveda, homoeopathy, yoga, naturopahty, acupressure, magnetotherapy, water-therapy, massage and aromatherapy etc and on all major ailments.

Dr. Rajeev Sharma is Medical Advisor to Ralson Remedies (a homoeopathic manufacturer), and Dixit Pharmacy (Ayurvedic Manufacturer), Sr. Medical Officer U.P. Govt. He has received several prizes for his outstanding achievements. He has been awarded the *Best Author prize in Hindi* by the Ministry of Health and Family Welfare, Government of India and *Sarjana Puraskar by U.P. Hindi Sansthan,* Lucknow. He has delivered talks on All India Radio and Total T.V. and lectures on Alternative Medicine in various Government and Non-government Organisations. He has written Advt. Scripts for the products of several companies.

He has established an institute through which you can get certificates by correspondence in Accupressure, Massage, Yoga,

Water Therapy, Diet Therapy, Naturopathy, Color Therapy and Reiki besides other paramedical courses.

He is providing literature on Personality Development and Life Style Management.

Dr. Rajeev Sharma is also a social activist. He has worked a lot against Addition and prevention of AIDS. He has worked for population and pollution control and human rights and has received the World Human Rights Promotion Award. His name has been published in *LIMCA BOOK OF RECORDS* 2005. He has developed a website too :- www.newkamasutra.com.

Contents

What is First Aid?

First aid is the immediate assistance or treatment given to someone injured or suddenly taken ill before the arrival of an ambulance, doctor or other appropriate qualified person. The person offering this help to a casualty must act calmly and with confidence, and above all must be willing to offer assistance whenever the need arises.

Being a First Aider

Most people can, by following the guidance given in this book, give useful and effective first aid. However, first aid is a skill based on knowledge, training, and experience. The term 'First Aider' is usually applied to someone who has completed a theoretical and practical instruction course, and passed a professionally supervised examination. A certificate is valid for only three years; to keep up to date, you must be re-examined after further training. Once qualified, you may volunteer for additional training to broaden the scope of your skills.

Aims of First Aid

- To preserve life.
- To limit worsening of the condition.
- To promote recovery.

The First Aider is

- Highly trained.
- Examined and regularly re-examined.
- Up-to-date knowledge and skill.

Being A First Aider

The first aid learned from a manual or course is not quite like reality. Most of us feel apprehensive when dealing with "the real thing". By facing up to these feelings, we are better able to cope with the unexpected.

Doing your part

First aid is not an exact science, and is thus open to human error. Even with appropriate treatment, and however hard you try, a casualty may not respond as hoped. Some conditions inevitably lead to death, even with the best medical care. If you do your best, your conscience can be clear.

Assessing risks

The golden rule is, "First do no harm", while applying the principle of "calculated risk". You should use the treatment that is most likely to be of benefit to a casualty, but do not use a doubtful treatment just for the sake of doing something.

The "Good Samaritan"

This principle supports those acting in an emergency (but not those who go beyond accepted boundaries). If you keep calm, and you follow the guidelines in this book, you need not fear any legal consequences.

Protecting the Casualty

To avoid cross-infection when giving first aid, if possible you should;

- avoid direct contact with body fluids where possible;

- wash your hands;
- wear protective gloves.

If gloves are unavailable, life saving treatment must be given.

Your Responsibilities as a First Aider

To assess a situation quickly and safely and summon appropriate help.

To protect casualties and others at the scene from possible danger. To identify, as far as possible, the injury or nature of the illness affecting a casualty.

To give each casualty early and appropriate treatment, treating the most serious conditions first.

To arrange for the casualty's removal to hospital, into the care of a doctor, or to his or her home.

To remain with a casualty until appropriate care is available.

To report your observations to those taking over of the casualty, and to give further assistance if required.

Prevent cross-infection between yourself and the casualty as much as possible.

Giving Care with Confidence

Every casualty needs to feel secure and in safe hands. You can create an air of confidence and assurance by:

- being in control, both of yourself and the problem;
- acting calmly and logically;
- being gentle, but firm, with your hands, and speaking to the casualty kindly, but purposefully.

Building up trust

Talk to the casualty throughout your examination and treatment.

- Explain what you are going to do.
- Try to answer questions honestly to allay fears as best you can. If you do not know the answer, say so.
- Continue to reassure the casualty even when your treatment is complete - find out about, the next-of-kin, or anyone else who should be contacted about the incident. Ask if you can help to make arrangements so that any responsibilities the casualty may have, such as collecting a child from school, can be taken care of.
- Do not leave someone whom you believe to be dying. Continue to talk to the casualty and hold his or her hand; never let the person feel alone.

Talking to relatives

The task of informing relatives of a death is usually the job of the police or the doctor on duty. However, you have to tell relatives or friends that someone is ill, or has been involved in an accident.

Always check that you are speaking to the right person first. Then explain, as simply and honestly as you can, what has happened, and, if appropriate, where the casualty has been taken. Do not be vague, or exaggerate; you may cause undue alarm. It is better to admit ignorance than to give misleading information.

Coping with children

Young children are extremely perceptive and will quickly detect any uncertainty on your part. Gain an injured or sick child's confidence by talking first to someone he or she trusts - a parent if possible. If the parent accepts you and believes you will help, this confidence will be conveyed to the child.

Always explain simply to a child what is happening and what you intend to do; do not talk over his or her head. You should not separate a child from his or her mother, father or other trusted person.

Looking after Yourself

It is important not to jeopardise your personal safety. Do not attempt heroic rescues in hazardous circumstances.

Coping with unpleasantness

The practice of first aid can be messy and smelly, and you may feel that you will not be able to cope with this. Such fears are common but usually groundless. First-aid training will bolster your self-reliance and confidence and will help you to control your emotions in a difficult situation.

Taking stock after an emergency

Assisting at an emergency is a stressful event, and you may suffer a "delayed reaction" some time afterwards. You may feel satisfaction or even elation, but it is common to be upset, particularly if the casualty was a stranger and you might not know the outcome of your efforts.

Above all, never reproach yourself, or bottle up your feelings. It often helps to talk over your experience with a friend, your doctor or your first-aid trainer.

You may worry about picking up infections from casualties. Often, simple measures such as washing your hands and wearing gloves will protect both you and the casualty from cross-infection.

However, there is a risk that blood-borne viruses, such as hepatitis B or C and HIV (which can lead to AIDS -Acquired Immune Deficiency Syndrome), may be spread by blood-to-blood contact.

These viruses can be transmitted only if an infected person's blood makes contact with a break in the skin, such as a cut or abrasion containing blood or blood products, of another person. No evidence exists of hepatitis or HIV being passed on during mouth-to-mouth resuscitation.

To prevent cross-infection, you should:

- always carry protective gloves;
- cover your own sores or skin wounds with a waterproof plaster;
- wear a plastic apron when dealing with large quantities of a casualty's body fluids and wear plastic glasses to protect your eyes against splashes;
- take care not to prick yourself with any needle found on or near the casualty, or to cut yourself from glass;
- if your eyes, nose or mouth or any wound on your skin is splashed by the casualty's blood, wash thoroughly with soap and water as soon as possible, and consult a doctor;
- use a mask or face shield for mouth-to-mouth ventilation if the casualty's mouth or nose is bleeding;
- dispose of blood and waste safely after treating the casualty.

Seeking Immunisation

First Aiders should seek medical advice on hepatitis B immunisation from their own doctors. If, after giving first aid, you are concerned that you have been in contact with infection of any sort, seek further medical advice.

Action at an Emergency

Effective first aid usually begins before any direct contact with the casualty, you should approach any incident with firmness, authority, and control in order to reassure the casualty and any bystanders. This is particularly important if there are many casualties, when a calm, systematic attitude on your part can help to prevent further injuries and enhance the survival of the casualties.

The principles of emergency first aid

Clear rules exist to ensure safety in hazardous situations and this chapter will make you aware of these. You will also learn how and when to alert the emergency services, understand which branch is appropriate to different emergencies, and be able to brief them clearly on their arrival.

First-AID Priorities

Assess the situation

- Observe what has happened quickly and calmly.
- Look for dangers to yourself and to the casualty.
- Never put yourself at risk.

Make the area safe

- Protect the casualty from danger.
- Be aware of your limitations.

Assess all casualties and give emergency first aid

- Assess each casualty to determine treatment priorities, and treat those with life-threatening conditions first.

Get help

- Quickly ensure that any necessary specialist help has been summoned and is on its way.

The Practice of First Aid

In most situations that require first aid, there will be no life-threatening danger. You will simply be assisting a conscious casualty; whose recovery from some minor injury or illness is not in doubt. In all cases, your aim is to work to a plan and discover what is wrong with the casualty, and to give prompt, correct treatment in a methodical way.

Assessing the situation

Before tending to a casualty, however, you must survey the whole scene. Your first responsibility is to make sure that the area is safe. Often hazards such as passing traffic can be dealt with simply, but where the danger is too great or too imminent, you may need to move the casualty even at the risk of aggravating the injury. Do this only if it is safe to approach the casualty: you cannot help others if you also become a casualty. Only when the casualty is safe can you begin to treat the illness or injury.

The First Aider Should

- Preserve life
- Pay strict attention to safety
- Follow the ABC of resuscitation
- Control any major bleeding
- Limit worsening of the condition
- Make a diagnosis of the injury or illness, if possible, by means of a thorough examination.
- Give priority to seriously injured casualties.

- Treat multiple injuries in order of priority dealing with life-threatening conditions first. Consider the possibility of "hidden" secondary conditions.
- Promote the casualty's recovery.
- Relieve any discomfort, pain or anxiety. Arrange for appropriate medical attention.

Initial Assessment

When you are sure, that it is safe to do so, quickly perform a brief examination of the casualty. This initial assessment is to check for any life-threatening conditions that need urgent first aid to preserve life.

You must perform the checks shown below before making a full diagnosis, and, if necessary, you should be prepared to carry out the appropriate steps to resuscitate the casualty first.

If you suspect that there may be head or neck injuries involved, move the casualty very carefully and only if it is absolutely necessary.

1. Sending for help

If you think it is needed, send for help promptly. Try to send someone else while you stay with the casualty, but ensure that they report back to you after making the call.

I. Check for consciousness

II. The casualty doctors doctors not respond when spoken to, he may be unconscious. Try to elicit a response.Be careful not to move the head or neck.

2. Open the airway

An unconscious casualty's airway may be blocked by the tongue falling back. Open the airway by tilting the head back.

3. Check for breathing

Once the casualty's airway is open, establish whether he is breathing. If so, place in the recovery position and if not then give two breaths.

4. Check for circulation

If the heart is beating, you should be able to feel a pulse in the neck or at the wrist. Check for a baby's pulse on the inside of the upper arm.

5. Check for bleeding

Severe loss of blood reduces the circulation to the vital organs, and can cause serious shock. Control serious bleeding as soon as breathing and pulse are established.

What to do Next?

As soon as you have established the condition of the casualty, take appropriate action, based on whether he is: unconscious, not breathing, and without a pulse or with a pulse.

Making a Diagnosis

Once you have completed your initial assessment and made sure that the casualty is out of immediate danger, you need to make a diagnosis; this often requires a thorough physical.

If diagnosis is made, on the basis of this history and clues to any medical condition, and symptoms and signs. Circumstances will determine how detailed your examination will be. In wet, cold conditions, when an ambulance is on its way, only serious injuries need attention - the priority is to keep the casualty warm and dry. If a conscious casualty can describe the symptoms, concentrate on treating those.

History

This is the full story of how the incident happened, how the injury was sustained, how the illness began and continued, including any previous conditions.

Question the casualty, but if he or she is unconscious, talk to any onlookers.

Witnesses can give useful information, but they can be unreliable, particularly if they are upset. Try to form a full picture of what took place. Take into account:

- when the casualty last had something – in eating or drinking;
- whether the casualty has any illness or is taking any medication;
- the amount of force involved and how it was applied to the body;
- the environment – was the casualty in a hot and stuffy, or cold room exposed to wind or rain;
- the casualty's age and state of health: a young, fit adult who trips may sprain a wrist, but an elderly lady who does the same is more likely to have broken his/her arm or hip;
- establish who the casualty is, and where he or she lives. Make a note of this information, including the time of injury and your examination.

External Clues

If the casualty is unable to co-operate or is unconscious, look through pockets and bags for clues (beware of syringes if you suspect drug abuse). There may be an appointment card for a hospital or clinic or a card indicating a history of allergy, diabetes or epilepsy. Horse-riders or cyclists may carry such a card in a riding hat or helmet.

Medication carried by the casualty may give valuable clues about the emergency. Medical warning items ("Medic-Alert" or an "SOS Talisman") may be worn as a locket, bracelet, medallion, or on a key ring; some contain medical information. Take care of any such item and return it to the casualty.

Symptoms and Signs

Every injury and illness manifests itself in distinctive ways that may help your diagnosis. These indications are divided into two groups: symptoms and signs. Some will be obvious, but others may be missed unless you examine the casualty thoroughly from head to toe. A conscious casualty should be examined, wherever possible, in the position found, or with any obvious injury comfortably supported; an unconscious casualty's airway must first be opened and secured. Do not remove clothing unnecessarily and do not leave the casualty exposed to cold conditions any longer than required.

Use your senses – look, listen, feel, and smell. Be quick and alert, but be thorough, and do not make unjustified assumptions. You should handle the casualty gently, but your touch must be firm enough to ensure that you feel any swelling or irregularity or detect a tender spot. Ask a conscious casualty to describe any sensations your touch causes.

Assessing Symptoms

Symptoms are sensations that the casualty experiences, and may be able to describe, if she is conscious. Ask if she has any abnormal sensations, if there is any pain, where it is felt, what type of pain it is, and how movement affects it. If the pain did not follow an injury, find out how and where it began. Severe pain in one place can mask a more serious, but less painful injury in another.

Ask if there are any other symptoms such as nausea, giddiness, heat, cold, weakness, or thirst. All symptoms should be assessed and confirmed, wherever appropriate, by an examination for signs of injury or illness.

Looking for Signs

Signs are details of a casualty's condition that you can see, feel, hear or smell. Many are obvious, but others may be discovered only during a thorough examination. Assess the casualty's level of response.

If he/she is unconscious or unable to Speak clearly, you may have to make a diagnosis purely on the circumstances i.e. incident, information obtained from onlookers and the signs you find.

Apply your senses

Look for bleeding, discolouration or deformity. Feel the strength and rhythm of the pulse and listen to the breathing.

Gently feel parts of the body that are painful, noting tenderness or variation in the alignment of a bone. Note if the casualty is unable to perform any normal function, such as moving a limb. Use your sense of smell to search for clues.

Symptoms and Signs of Injury or Illness

The casualty may tell you of these symptoms –

• Pain • Anxiety • Heat • Cold • Loss of normal movement • Loss of sensation • Abnormal sensation • Thirst • Nausea • Tingling Faintness • Stiffness • Momentary unconsciousness • Weakness • Memory loss • Dimness • Sensation of broken bone.

You may see these signs

• Anxiety and painful expression • Unusual chest movement • Sweating • Wounds • Bleeding from orifices • Response to touch Response to speech • Bruising • Abnormal skin colour • Muscle spasm Swelling • Deformity • Foreign bodies • Needle marks • Vomit Incontinence • Containers and other circumstantial evidence.

You may feel these signs

• Dampness • Abnormal body temperature • Tenderness to touch or pressure • Swelling • Deformity • Irregularity • Grating bone ends.

You may hear these signs

• Noisy or distressed breathing • Groaning • Sucking sounds (chest Injury) • Response to touch • Response to speech • Grating bone (crepitus) • Solvents or glue.

You may smell these signs; remember to smell the casualty's breath

• Acetone • Alcohol • Burning • Gas or fumes incontinence • Cannabis.

Examining a Casualty

A detailed examination of the casualty should be undertaken only after taking any vital action needed. You may need to move or remove clothing, but ensure that, at every stage of your examination, you do not move the casualty more than is absolutely-necessary. Always start at the head and work down; the "top-to-toe" routine is both easily remembered and thorough.

Top-to-Toe Survey

1. Run your hands carefully over the scalp to feel for bleeding, swelling or depression, that may indicate a possible fracture. Be careful not to move any casualty who you think may have injured her neck, especially if she is unconscious.
2. Speak clearly to the casualty in both ears to see if she responds or if she can hear. Look for blood or clear fluid (or a mixture of both) coming from either ear. These may be signs of damage inside the skull.
3. Examine both eyes, noting if they are open, the size of the pupils, whether they are equal in size, and whether they react to light (each pupil should shrink, when light falls on it). Look for any-foreign body, blood, or bruising in the whites of the eyes.
4. Check the nose for the same signs as in the ears. Look for blood or clear fluid (or a mixture of both) coming from either nostril. Any of these might indicate damage inside the skull.

5. Record the rate, depth, and nature (easy or difficult, noisy or quiet) of breathing. Note any odour in breath. Look and feel inside the mouth for anything that might endanger the airway. If dentures are intact and fit firmly, leave them in place. Look for any wound in the mouth or irregularity in the line of the teeth. Examine the lips for burns.
6. Note the colour, temperature, and state of the skin: is it pale, flushed or grey-blue (cyanosis); is it hot or cold, dry or damp? For example, pale, cold, sweaty skin suggests shock; a flushed, hot face suggests heatstroke or fever. A blue tinge indicates lack of oxygen; look for this especially in the lips, ears, and face.
7. Loosen clothing around the neck, and look for any warning medallion, or hole in the windpipe left by a surgical operation. Run your fingers gently along the spine from the base, of the skull downwards as far as possible, without disturbing the casualty's position, checking for irregularity, swelling or tenderness.
8. Ask the casualty to breathe deeply; and note whether the chest expands, easily, and equally on both sides. Gently feel the ribcage for any deformity, irregularity, tenderness or a grating sensation in breathing. Observe whether breathing causes the casualty any pain or discomfort. Look for signs of bleeding from any wounds.
9. Gently feel along both the collar bones and the shoulders for any deformity, irregularity or tenderness.
10. Check the movements of elbows, wrists and fingers by asking the casualty to bend and straighten the arm at the joints. Check that the casualty can feel normally with her fingers and there are no abnormal sensations in the limbs. Note the colour in the fingers, whether they are pale or grey-blue, as this indicate a problem with the circulation. Look for any needle marks on the forearms, or a warning bracelet. Take the pulse at the wrist or neck.

11. If there is any sign of impairment of movement or loss of sensation in the limbs, do not move the casualty to examine the spine. Otherwise, gently pass your hand under the hollow of the back and feel along the spine without disturbing the casualty, checking for swelling and tenderness.
12. Gently feel the front of the abdomen for evidence of bleeding, and to identify any rigidity or tenderness of the muscular wall.
13. Feel both sides of the hips, and gently move the pelvis to look for signs of fracture. Note any incontinence or bleeding from orifices.
14. Ask the casualty to raise each leg and turn, and to move her ankles and knees. Look and feel for bleeding, swelling, deformity or tenderness.
15. Check movement and feeling in all the toes. Look at their colour to indicate a circulatory disorder or cold injury.

Removing Clothing

You may have to remove clothing to make a thorough examination, to obtain an accurate diagnosis, or to give the casualty appropriate treatment. This should be done with the minimum of disturbance to the casualty. Only remove as much clothing as is strictly necessary; try to maintain privacy for the casualty and prevent exposure to cold conditions as far as possible. Do not damage clothing unless it is absolutely necessary and, where you can, cut along the seams or sleeves.

Removing Footwear

Support the ankle and carefully remove the shoe. Long boots may need to be slit down the back seam with a sharp knife.

Removing Socks

If socks cannot be pulled off gently, lift each one away from the leg with your fingers and cut the sock with scissors.

Removing Trousers

Gently pull up the trouser leg to expose the calf and knee, or pull trousers down from the waist to reveal the thigh.

Removing a Sweater

1. Carefully remove the casualty's uninjure arm from its sleeve
2. Ease the garment over the casualty's head, without disturbing the injured arm, if possible.
3. Support the injured arm and slip off the other sleeve of the garment.

Removing a Coat or Shirt

1. Unbutton the garment, and pull it off the casualty's shoulders.
2. Remove the uninjured arm from its sleeve first, and pull the garment round to the injured side.
3. Support the injured arm and ease, the garment of the arm, keeping the arm straight if possible.

Removing Protective Helmets

A protective helmet, is best left on, and should be removed only if absolutely necessary (for example, a lull-lace helmet that encloses the head and lace may prevent you from performing artificial ventilation). Any helmet should always, if possible, be removed by the casualty. Ideally, two people are required to remove a helmet so that the casualty's head and neck are constantly supported. The casualty's head should also be carefully aligned with the spine in the neutral position. If it is necessary to remove the helmet.

For an Open-face Helmet or Riding Hat

DO NOT remove the helmet, unless it is absolutely necessary.

1. Unfasten the buckle, or cut through the chinstrap.
2. If the helmet or hat has sides, grip it from above, and force the sides of the helmet apart to take pressure off the casualty's head. Gently lift the helmet upwards and backwards to remove it.

For a Full-face Helmet

DO NOT remove the helmet unless it is absolutely necessary.

1. Undo or cut the straps. Working from the base of the helmet, ease the lingers of both your hands underneath the rim. Support the neck with one hand and hold the lower jaw firmly.

2. Ask a helper, working from above, to tilt the helmet backwards (try not) to move the head at all) and gently lift the front clear of the casualty's chin.
3. Continue, to support the neck and jaw. Ask your helper to tilt the helmet forwards slightly so that it will pass over the base of the skull, and then to lift it straight off the casualty's head.

Treatment and Aftercare

Treat each condition methodically and calmly in order of priority. Reassure the casualty, and listen to what, he or she has to say. Do not keep questioning the casualty, do not let people crowd around, and avoid moving him or her unnecessarily.

Treatment priorities

- Follow the ABC of resuscitation.
- Maintain a clear airway and breathing; if unconscious, place in the recovery position.
- Control bleeding. Treat large wounds and burns.
- Immobilise bone and joint injuries.
- Give, appropriate treatment for other injuries and conditions.
- Check airway, breathing, and pulse regularly and deal with any problem immediately.

Arranging appropriate aftercare

Ascertain whether the casualty needs medical treatment and, if so, what is needed. If you require help, send someone else, if possible, in the event that the casualty's condition alters or worsens. Stay with the casualty until help arrives. According to your assessment of the casualty, you may:

- call a doctor for advice;
- call an ambulance or arrange transport to hospital;
- pass care of the casualty to a doctor, nurse or ambulance crew;
- take dying casualty to a nearby house or shelter to await medical help;

- allow the casualty to go home, accompanied if possible – ask someone to be at home to meet him or her, or, if you can, arrange this;
- advise the casualty to see a doctor.

DO NOT allow to go home a casualty who has been unconscious, had severe breathing difficulty or signs of shock. Stay with him or her until help arrives.

DO NOT give anything by mouth to any casualty who may have internal injuries or otherwise need hospital care.

Care of Personal Belongings

If you have to search a casualty's belongings for identification or clues to his condition, make sure that you do so in front of a reliable witness. Take care of any-clothing or property, and ensure that it accompanies the casualty to hospital, or is handed over to the police. Make sure that someone accepts responsibility for contacting the casualty's family.

Passing on Information

Having summoned medical aid, try to make notes on the incident and the condition of the casualty so that you can pass on all the information you have gathered. The observation chart overleaf, which is recommended for use by all three Voluntary Aid Societies, will enable you to note your observations of the casualty's condition, such as pulse, breathing, and level of response, clearly and at intervals of ten minutes. If the casualty is in a critical condition, record these observations more frequently.

Make a brief written report to accompany your observations. A record of the timing of events is particularly valuable to medical personnel. Note carefully, for example, the length of a period of unconsciousness, the duration of a fit, the time of any changes in the casualty's condition, and the time of any intervention or treatment.

If possible, stay with the casualty until help arrives, or accompany him or her to the hospital, so that you can hand over your notes personally.

Making a report

Your report should include:

- The casualty's name, and address;
- History of the accident or illness;
- A brief description of any injuries;
- Any unusual behaviour;
- Any treatment given, and when;
- Breathing, pulse, and level of response.

The Use of Medication

Medication within first aid is largely confined to relieving general aches and pains, and is generally limited to helping a casualty to take paracetamol, as described in the relevant sections of this book.

A wide range of medications may be bought over the counter without a doctor's prescription, and you may know and have used many of them. However, when treating a casualty, you must not buy or borrow medication to administer it yourself, even if the casualty has forgotten his or her own medication or you have the type they may normally expect to use.

If you administer or advise any medication other than those stipulated in this manual when giving first aid, the casualty may be put at risk, and you could find yourself facing legal or civil action as a consequence

If the necessary medication is not available, seek expert medical treatment. The only exception to this principle occurs where there are clear protocols laid down by an employer or voluntary organisation. Such protocols allow trained staff or members to adminster medication in specific circumstances, such as antidotes to industrial poisons.

Whenever medication is taken, it is essential to ensure that:

- it is appropriate for the condition;
- it is not out of date;
- it is taken as advised;
- any precautions are strictly followed;
- the recommended dose is not exceeded whatever the circumstances;
- a detailed record is kept of all medication administered.

Observation Chart

The information from this chart will be very valuable when decisions are taken about further treatment:

- use a photocopy of it to record your observations while waiting for help;
- tick the appropriate boxes;
- update them at ten-minute intervals;
- send the completed chart, and any notes, with the casualty when he or she leaves your care.

Date .... Casualty's Name ....

Time of observation (10-minute intervals)		10	20	30	40	50	60
Eyes Observe for reaction while testing other responses	Open spontaneously						
	Open to speech						
	Open to painful stimulus						
	No Response						
Movement Apply painful stimulus pinch ear lobe or skin on back of hand	Obeys Commands						
	Responds to painful stimulus						
	No response						
Speech when testing responses, speak clearly and directly, close to casualty's ear.	Responds sensibly to questions						
	Seems confused						
	Uses inappropriate words						
	Incomprehensible sounds						
Pulse (beats per minute) Take pulse at wrist or at neck on adult; at inner arm on baby. Note rate, and whether beats are weak (w) or strong (s), regular (.reg) or irregular (irreg.)	Over 110						
	101-110						
	90-100						
	80-90						
	71-80						
	61-70						
	Below 01						
Breathing (breaths per minute) Note: rate, and whether breathing is quiet (q) or noisy (n) easy (e) or difficult (diff).	Over 40						
	31-40						
	21-30						
	11-20						
	Below 11						

Effects of Excessive Cold and Heat

Frostbite: An exposed extremity – the nose, ears, fingers or toes – goes cold and very pale, becomes stiff and painful, turns numb and may eventually be paralysed.

Cold exhaustion: The victim is cold, wet and tired. As body temperature falls cold exhaustion sets in. Speech begins to slurr, the victim shivers and has cramps, his vision is disturbed and he begins to stumble.

Severe hypothermia: If the exposure continues, the body becomes very cold (25 degrees Centigrade) and breathing slows and becomes shallow. Eventually core temperature drops to 20 degrees Centigrade and the victim dies.

Groups liable to severe hypothermia

1. Mountaineering and hiking expeditions
2. Sailing parties-especially after capsizing
3. Old people without adequate home heating
4. Very young children who are not properly dressed and cared for
5. Drug addicts and alcoholics who sleep rough
6. Others who might undergo prolonged unconsciousness, e.g. diabetics and epileptics

Effects of excessive heat

Local burns: Prolonged exposure to the sun's ultra-violet rays can bring severe burns to any uncovered part of the body.

Heat exhaustion: In a hot climate heat is lost by evaporation of sweat from the skin. If this is excessive the body will run short of salt and water and this may be followed by vomiting and diarrhoea.

Temperature usually remains close to normal, but the victim of heat exhaustion will be restless and at cramps.

Heat stroke: If the climate is hot and very humid little heat can be lost from the body by sweating. Core and surface temperatures therefore rise rapidly and this produces a headache and dizziness. The skin remains hot, dry and flushed and consciousness is rapidly lost.

Step by Step

Frostbite

Do not rub the affected area or reheat it rapidly.

Warm slowly using another part of the body if possible. Cover the nose or ears with the palm of the hand. Warm hands under the armpits and wrap the feet together in a blanket.

Cold exhaustion

Any expedition should be properly organised, planned and adequately supplied with wind and rain-proof clothing, shelter, energy-giving rations, flares, a large polythene bag, etc. Every member of the group should be fit and carry no more than one-third his own weight up to a maximum of 18 kilograms.

Severe hypothermia

If the victim of severe hypothermia is rewarmed rapidly, the blood vessels in the skin will dilate (enlarge) and draw blood supplies away from vital organs such as the brain. It is therefore essential that those suffering from severe hypothermia be reheated slowly by one or two blankets. Medical help should be urgently sought. If breathing or pulse stops, start immediate mouth to mouth resuscitation or external cardiac compression.

Do's

Rest: This is essential to overcoming exhaustion Insulation: The victim should be wrapped up in a warm blanket or sleeping bag and his head covered over.

Shelter: A tent or wind break such as a polythene sheet should be put up to reduce the victim's heat loss.

Food: If the victim is conscious he should be given warm, sweet drinks.

Rescue: Remove to base camp by the most comfortable method available.

At Base Camp: Reheat the victim rapidly by immersing the whole body in a hot bath (maximum temperature: 45 degrees Centigrade), get medical help.

Heat exhaustion: Move the casulty to shade.

Add ½ teaspoon of salt to a glass of water and feed to the victim. This will help replace the lost salt and fluids. Repeat the action but be careful not to administer too much salt as this will only make the victim ill and so aggravate the problem.

Heat stroke: The main aim here is to cool the victim. This should be done as follows:

- Remove to the shade
- Provide ventilation if possible (with a fan, etc.)
- Wrap in a damp sheet
- Seek medical help.

If Breathing Stops

Blocked airways: The airways may be blocked at any point. The most important sites are the pharynx (back of the mouth and nose) and the larynx. The pharynx may be blocked by the tongue, false teeth, vomit or blood. The larynx may be blocked by tight contraction of the vocal cords due to poisonous gases or inhaled material such as peanuts or fishbones.

Paralysed breathing mechanism: The brain usually sends messages through the spinal cord and then the nerves to supply the muscles which move the chest wall and diaphragm. The brain may be damaged by an accident or a stroke, for example. The spinal cord may be injured by a broken neck, the nerves may be paralysed by poliomyelitis, or the chest wall may be unable to move because it is trapped by a heavy weight or because the ribs are badly broken. In any of these cases, breathing may be stopped.

How do I know when breathing has stopped ?

Look closely at the victim's chest. If it is not moving up and down and there is no movement of air in and out of the mouth, he has stopped breathing. The victim will turn blue and his pulse (heart beat) will gradually weaken.

What emergency action should I take ?

Clear airways: Breathing may be stopped by an obstruction in the airways. Remove any false or broken teeth, spit, phlegm, vomit, etc.

Extend neck and pull the jaw forward: When the victim is lying on his back with his head in the normal position, the tongue blocks the airways. Extending the neck and pulling the jaw forward keeps the top part of the airway open and allows air to pass through.

Pinch the nose: Because the nose and mouth are connected by an air passage, it is necessary to keep the nose closed when blowing air through the mouth into the lungs. If the nose were left open, air would escape through it and not enter the lungs where it is needed. In the same way, if the rescuer uses the mouth to nose method of resuscitation, the victim's mouth must be kept closed if it is to work.

Open the mouth and apply mouth to mouth resuscitation: The victim is now ready to have air blown into his lungs. Keep the neck extended and the jaw pulled forward, pinch the nose and apply your mouth to the victim's, forming an airtight seal. Blow into the mouth-watch the chest. Does it rise? If not, check the airways for obstructions.

If it does rise, repeat the action two more times. This fills the lungs with air and gives you time to check that the pulse is strong; confirm that the victim is still not breathing.

If the pulse is strong and he is not breathing, continue mouth to mouth resuscitation, inflating the chest about 15 times a minute. Resuscitation should be continued until the victim begins breathing naturally again, or you are exhausted, or a doctor asks you to stop.

Step by Step

- Extending the neck
- Pinching the nose and opening the mouth
- Mouth to mouth resuscitation
- Blow into the mouth and watch the rise and fall of chest.

Obstruction of airways

Produced by false teeth, a loose tooth, peanuts or some other material stuck in an airway, this usually results in violent efforts to breathe and is accompanied by a great deal of noise from the airways. Treatment is aimed at dislodging the foreign body. A child should be turned upside down and shaken until the foreign body is removed. An adult should be bent over the knee and hit on the back until the obstruction has cleared away.

●

Bleeding

The arteries which lead from the heart are strong muscular and elastic tubes which contain blood under high pressure. Veins which go to the heart contain blood at low pressure. Between the arteries and veins are many microscopic tubes called capillaries. Bleeding can occur from any of these three types of vessels.

Each type of vessel bleeds in a different way:

Arterial bleeding occurs in spurts of blood in time with the heart beat.

Venous bleeding is a strong, steady flow.

Capillary bleeding is a slow, steady flow which quickly stops.

How the body stops bleeding?

When the skin is cut blood vessels are severed and bleeding follows. When this happens the blood vessels tighten up or contract, blood clots, and if much blood is lost, blood pressure falls. In these three ways blood loss is reduced.

Finding the pulses and pressure points

Each time the heart beats the blood pressure increases and a 'pulse' can be felt in the arteries. This pulse can be taken best where the artery can be pressed against a bone (at the pressure points).

Neck or carotid pulse:

Located at the point of the triangle between the shaded muscle which runs from the ear to the collar bone and the muscles covering the voice box (larynx) and the windpipe (trachea).

Wrist or radial pulse:

Can be found at the thumb side of the wrist in the position where the watch strap is usually worn. This is not a pressure point because the hand is also supplied by another artery.

Arm or brachial pulse:

Felt halfway down the inside of the arm between the bands of muscles above and below the arm bone. A nerve runs along this artery and if it is rolled on the bone it will produce a tingling sensation in the arm and little finger.

Thigh or femoral pulse:

Positioned halfway between the centre of the pubic bone and the front of the hip bone. This point is just on the inside of the leg below the groin skin crease.

When light pressure is applied to the artery, the pulse can be felt and counted, and have its strength measured. The normal pulse is between 60 to 90 beats a minute and should feel full and strong. Locate the pulses on yourself and practise how to find them quickly. If heavy pressure is applied to these sites, the arteries will be pushed against the bone and no blood will flow through. This may be used to control bleeding in a site supplied by that particular artery.

Internal bleeding

Several important organs such as the liver, spleen and kidneys are protected by the lower ribs. If these are broken the jagged ends of the ribs may puncture the tissues and cause serious internal bleeding. Broken bones and other damaged organs may also bleed. Often the only external signs of internal bleeding may be the development of shock (see signs of shock below) and/or the following:

- Vomiting or coughing up blood
- Passing blood in the urine
- Swelling of a limb around a broken bone
- Bruising over the lower ribs

External bleeding

This may happen if the skin is lacerated (torn with ragged edges), incised (cut with smooth edges like a razor slash), or stabbed. There would have to be a severe loss of blood before the victim's life was endangered, but even a little blood can look a lot if you are not used to dealing with it. The First-Aider is in a good position to deal with any of these and to control or stop external bleeding.

What is shock?

When the blood does not circulate properly to the tissues, they become deprived of oxygen and other essential foodstuffs. The victim is then said to be 'shocked' or 'in shock'. This poor circulation of blood may be due to:

Loss of blood: e.g. internal bleeding, external bleeding

Loss of fluid: e.g. from burns from severe vomiting or severe diarrhoea

Loss of pumping power from the heart: e.g. heart attacks, heart failure

Following a severe fright or severe pain: e.g. burst stomach ulcer after a serious accident.

Fainting

This is a temporary and very mild form of poor blood circulation to the brain. The person who has fainted usually falls to the ground, sweats, and has a fast pulse. Nothing needs to be done except perhaps to loosen tight clothing and to raise the legs. The victim will recover rapidly on his own.

A dirty wound

A wound is a breach in the protective layer covering the body. Germs such as bacteria and viruses enter the body through it and cause infections. This risk of serious complications is much greater when the wound is dirty or left open to the air. Dirty wounds should be washed with clean water or with a dilute solution of antiseptic, dressed and bandaged. A doctor should see any victim with a dirty wound because antibiotic and anti-tetanus injections may be needed.

Step by Step

External bleeding

Lie the victim down

Loosen tight clothing and expose the bleeding part.

ABC of shock

It is important to be able to recognise shock. The victim in shock may show any or all of the following signs:

- Anxious and trembling
- Blueness of the lips and paleness of the skin
- Cold clammy skin
- Dryness of the mouth
- Eyesight blurred and concentration poor
- Fast pulse

A victim in shock needs careful treatment: Tight clothing should be loosened and crowds should be moved away to allow the injured person to breath and relieve his anxiety. The victim must be laid flat to improve circulation to the brain. The legs should be raised to draw all available blood into the important part of the body and improve the circulation.

Shock occasionally produces difficulty in breathing. If this happens prop the victim up. The victim in shock should never be given anything to drink (water or alcohol, etc.) because an emergency operation may be necessary.

Apply direct pressure to the wound using:

- Dressings
- Bandages
- Clean handkerchiefs
- Tissues

Fresh newspapers, etc.

Raise the wounded part to lower the blood pressure in this area. Bandage the dressings in place. If bleeding does not stop apply more dressings. If this is not sufficient apply pressure to the Pressure (pulse) Point for a maximum of 15 minutes. Pressure can be re-applied after allowing one minute for the circulation to reach the limb. Arrange medical help as necessary. Check for pulse and general condition.

Tourniquets: These are tight bands tied around the limb often used in the past to prevent bleeding, but it is no longer recommended because it also restricts the return of blood to the heart through the veins and, if left in place for more than 15 minutes, may cause limbs to become gangrenous (dead).

Internal bleeding

Lie the victim down, loosen tight clothing, raise the legs and check his general condition. Get medical help as quickly as possible and try to comfort him.

Ear Canal

Wading from the ear canal may be produced by a serious skull injury by poking the ear. The First-Aider should do nothing other than lie ear with a pad to reduce infection and get medical help.

Nose

When hit or picked the nose, it usually bleeds and this is best treated by direct pressure. Pinch the nose between your finger and thumb. Sit the victim forward with his head over a sink-about ten minutes should be sufficient.

Gum

A bleeding tooth socket may be treated by placing a wad of cotton wool, tissues or handkerchief over the bleeding area, but not in the tooth socket, and having the victim bite down on the dressing. After ten minutes the bleeding will usually have stopped and the dressing can be removed. The victim should then sit upright and should neither walk nor lie down.

Lip, tongue or cheek

The bleeding part should be grasped between a dressing and local pressure applied for approximately ten minutes.

Scalp

When the scalp is wounded there is always the possibility that the skull underneath is broken. For this reason it is advisable not to apply direct pressure but place a ring pad on the wound instead. This will protect an underlying fracture.

Palm of hand

A dressing should be placed in the palm and the hand closed tightly. The hand should then be raised and supported in a sling.

Varicose veins

If a varicose vein suddenly bursts the loss of blood may be torrential. Prompt action is essential. Lie the victim down, apply direct pressure to the bleeding vein and elevate the leg.

Foreign bodies in the wound

Where a foreign body such as glass or a fish hook remains in a bleeding wound, it should be removed only if it can be done easily. If the foreign body is stuck leave it in position. No direct pressure can be applied in this case and a ring pad must be used.

Bruises

These are often called contusions and are a form of internal bleeding just under the skin (a black eye is one example). There is rarely very serious bleeding and continuous bleeding should be treated with a cold compress or ice pack.

Penetrating wound

Chest : A stab wound in the chest may cause serious internal bleeding which will require urgent hospital treatment. It may also collapse the lung by allowing air to enter the space between the lung and the chest wall. This may partially be prevented by applying a dressing over the wound.

Abdomen: This may also result in severe internal bleeding or cause serious damage to an internal organ. Medical help must be sought urgently.

●

When does the Heart stop?

When the heart stops the victim is said to have a 'cardiac arrest'. This can be caused by:

When breathing stops ('ventilatory arrest') Following strokes, Poisoning Electric shock or Heart attack, Severe injury.

Feel the carotid pulse

Within a few seconds of the heart stopping the victim loses consciousness and the skin looses its colour and becomes white often with a tinge of blue around the lips. The pulse may slow down until at last it disappears completely, or stop abruptly. The pupils widen. In cases of suspected cardiac arrest check the neck or carotid pulse to see if the heart is still beating. This pulse can be felt in the triangle between the windpipe and the shaded muscle which runs between the bone beneath the ear and the collar bone. Do not use the wrist pulse because it may be difficult to find and if it is weak it cannot be felt even though the heart is still beating. If the heart does not restart, the victim will soon stop breathing and the brain will be permanently damaged by the lack of blood supply in about three minutes. It is therefore vital that the heart quickly begins pumping again or that the blood keeps flowing to the brain. Only the person on the spot can do this within the time limit and the First Aider is in a unique position to save a life in such a situation by external cardiac compression.

External cardiac compression

External cardiac compression is the name given to the artificial way of keeping the blood circulating to the vital organs and particularly the brain. The heart lies between the breast bone (sternum) at the front of the body and the back bone (vertebral column) at the back. Lie the victim face up on a hard surface like the floor and not a soft bed. This will keep the victim rigid. The breast bone can then be pressed down towards the backbone. The heart will be compressed and blood squeezed out into the circulatory system.

External cardiac compression with mouth to mouth resuscitation

When the heart stops, the brain is deprived of oxygen with the result that the part of the brain which controls breathing quickly stops working and the victim stops breathing. Likewise, if the victim stops breathing, the heart will not receive oxygen and will not beat properly. If these two situations occur at the same time both external cardiac compression and mouth to mouth resuscitation will be needed to save the victim.

If two people are available then one should concentrate on giving mouth to mouth resuscitation, checking the pupil size (are they wide or narrow), and feeling the neck pulse. The other should carry on with the external cardiac compression. It is important that the chest should not be inflated at the same time as the heart is compressed. A rhythm of one inflation of the chest followed by five external cardiac compressions repeated ten times a minute produces the best results. If only one person is available to give first aid many precious minutes can be wasted by switching from external cardiac compression to giving mouth to mouth resuscitation. The best method is to inflate the chest twice and then compress the heart 15 times. This should be done at the rate of four times a minute.

	One person	**Two persons**
Lungs Heart Frequency	Two chest inflations followed by 15 cardiac compressions repeated 4 times a minute.	One chest inflation followed by 5 cardiac compressions repeated 10 times a minute

Step by Step

Feel the carotid pulse

This will confirm that the heart has stopped. Quickly place the victim on a hard surface and kneel beside him.

Strike the lower breastbone sharply

This should be done with the side of the hand. It may shock the heart into restarting. Feel the pulse. If the heart is not beating then start external cardiac compression.

Compress the heart

Place the heel of the hand two-thirds of the way down the breastbone and press downwards. Considerable pressure is needed because the breastbone must be moved about four to five centimetres each time. This should be repeated about 60 times a minute.

How do I know the heart is working?

The pupils in the eye will become smaller some colour will return to the face a strong carotid pulse will be felt with each compression

How long do I carry on?

until the heart starts beating by itself again

OR

an ambulance man, nurse or doctor, or more experienced first-aider tells you to stop

OR

you feel completely worn out.

The victim is not dead until you have given up trying to resuscitate him.

External cardiac compression in babies and young children

The hearts of infants are much smaller than adults and must decompressed with less force. For instance, a baby of less than one year old needs about 120 compressions each minute. But it takes very little force to move a baby's breastbone and one thumb is all that is needed to produce the necessary pressure. It is also important to realise that an infant's heart is much higher in the chest and that the breast bone must be pressed in the middle and not over the lower half. •

Different Pains

Toothache

Treatment for toothache is simple: rest, avoid the extremes of hot and cold, keep the mouth warm and go to the dentist or doctor.

Earache

Low pressure outside: Lessen the pressure on the middle ear by swallowing.

This is produced by pressure which stretches part of the inner ear. It can be caused by high pressure – for example, when diving and swimming under water or coming into land in aeroplane: low pressure (i.e. taking off an aeroplane) can also cause some pain in the ear. Inflammation of the ear can also cause painful stretching of the membrane in the inner ear. All earaches are dealt with by equalising pressure on both sides of the ear drum.

High pressure outside: Increase the pressure on the middle ear by blowing air into the ear. Hold the nose and blow the cheeks out.

Pressure increase caused by inflammation: In this case pressure cannot be reduced because the tube leading from the inside of the ear to the back of the throat is blocked. Take the victim to the doctor.

Black eye

If someone is hit in the eye bruising (light bleeding into the tissues) and swelling will develop. The bleeding stretches the tissues and causes pain. Swelling can be reduced by applying an ice-pack to the eye. As swelling goes down the pain is lessened.

Cramp

When a muscle tightens and becomes hard it is painful. This pain is called muscle cramp, or simply, cramp. The way to get rid of a cramp is to break the tightness of the muscle by stretching it. Calf muscles that are cramped should be stretched by pulling the foot back and straightening the knee. The tightness and pain will quickly disappear. Fingers or toes that are cramped should be straightened and pulled back. Sometimes cramp is caused by lack of salt, especially if the weather is hot and sticky. You sweat heavily and the body loses too much salt. In this case, put ½ a teaspoonful of salt in a large tumbler of water and drink it.

Stitch

This is the name given to cramps of the belly and chest wall. They are usually caused by strenuous exercise such as running. The way to ease the pain is to stretch the muscles by rubbing the painful part.

Winding

A sharp blow in the 'stomach' may hit the major nerve centre in the abdomen – the solar plexus – and cause fainting and pain. The victim should be placed in a comfortable position and tight clothes unfastened. If the victim is only partially conscious, put him in the recovery position.

Hiccups

This is due to sudden contraction of the diaphragm which is a sheet of muscle separating the chest and abdomen. Thinking about it often makes it much worse. Distract the victim by having him sip water or take slow deep breaths. If the hiccups don't stop it may distress the person so much that a doctor will be needed.

•

Foreign Bodies

When an object which does not belong to the body such as a safety pin, peanut or an insect gets into part of the body it is called a foreign body. It may produce pain, bleeding or irritation. In most cases it is best to remove the object, but if this cannot be done without causing further damage to the victim, leave it in position and call a doctor.

In the eye

Foreign body on the exposed part of the eye: Grit or insects often get into the eyes and cause irritation, redness and watering. Gently wipe the foreign body out with a wisp of cotton wool or the folded corner of a clean handkerchief.

Foreign body under the lower eyelid: In this case pull the eyelid away and remove the foreign body in the same way described above.

Foreign body under the upper eyelid: The upper eyelid cannot be easily pulled away from the eye because it contains a tough inner layer of cartilage. It may be possible to remove the foreign body by placing the upper lid over the lower lid in such a way that the object comes off on the lower lid. If this fails, then place a hairgrip or matchstick along the top of the upper lid, flip the lid over and remove the foreign body.

Acids and other caustic substances: If one of these gets into the eye it should be removed rapidly by flooding with water.

In the ear

At the bottom of the tube which leads from the outer ear there is a delicate membrane called the ear drum. This can be damaged by a foreign body especially if someone tries to poke the object out. Pour lukewarm water into the ear-this may remove the foreign body. If unsuccessful, see a doctor. Under no circumstance should the foreign body be poked about with a matchstick, tweezers, hairgrip, etc.

In the throat

Fishbones, peanuts and other pieces of food are the usual culprits in this case. The foreign body may irritate the throat and produce a tightening of the vocal cord muscles. This causes noisy and difficult breathing and the victim can easily suffocate. Help the victim to cough up the foreign body. This can be done by a sharp slap on the back between the shoulder blades.

In the stomach

Occasionally, a young child may swallow a nail or safety pin. This may puncture the wall of the stomach or guts. Get medical help immediately. Do not give anything by mouth as an operation may be needed to remove the unwanted object.

DEALING WITH DISASTER

What to do first

When there are several victims or several injuries and action is needed you must choose which job to do first. There are four conditions which need immediate treatment and they should be done in the following order:

1. When the heart has stopped-do external cardiac compression
2. When breathing has stopped-start mouth to mouth resuscitation
3. When an artery is bleeding-stop the flow of blood with pressure
4. When the casualty is unconscious-place in the recovery position

Quick action is the key to saving life. Because you cannot do everything at once, leave minor injuries and concentrate on life-saving jobs.

Poison

A poison is a substance which is harmful to the body. If too much of almost anything is taken it may be poisonous. Poisons include:

Gases such as coal gas containing carbon monoxide, sulphur dioxide, etc.

Tablets: such as heart or nerve pills

Liquids: such as weedkillers, bleaches and acids

Plants: such as toadstools, laburnum, etc.

Usually taken into the mouth, poisons pass through the gullet or oesophagus and into the stomach. Two tubes pass downwards from the back of the mouth; the one at the front is the windpipe or trachea; at the back is the gullet. The stomach is a baglike enlargement of the gut which acts like a reservoir for food. Digestion starts here.

Effects of poison

Corrosive poisons such as acids and weedkillers usually burn the mouth, gullet and stomach as they are swallowed. All poisons have a powerful effect on the nervous system either exciting (as in the case of amphetamines) or depressing it (as in the case of barbiturates or sleeping tablets).

Stages of consciousness

Any person who has been poisoned may lapse into unconsciousness. Progress of unconscious victims is measured in the following four stages:

i. Fully conscious: awake and can talk sensibly
ii. Drowsy: awake at times but seems to dose off. Speech is slurred

iii. Stupor: will wake up only if severe pain is inflicted
iv. Coma: cannot be woken up

How can I help?

The First Aider has a special opportunity in the case of poisons as only swift action will save the life of the victim.

If the victim is conscious, is breathing without difficulty and has a satisfactory pulse, check whether the poison has caused any corrosion. This will be indicated by burns in or around the mouth.

Provided that there is no corrosion, induce vomiting by: - forcing two fingers down the victim's throat

OR

making him drink a mixture of salt and water

OR

a solution of mustard and water

OR

Ipecac syrup

If the victim's mouth is burnt, dilute the poison with water or milk to neutralize its corrosive effects. Treat any pain caused by the corrosion with something soothing such as ice cream or olive oil.

Do not make the victim vomit as this will only result in the same corrosive poison burning the mouth and gullet again. It could even burn through the gullet wall and this would be a very serious complication.

Both corrosive and non-corrosive poisons may be treated with activated charcoal. This substance consists of fine, specially prepared charcoal particles which are mixed with water and swallowed. This prevents the absorption of a wide variety of poisonous substances.

Intentional overdose

Self-poisoning is an important and not uncommon cause of serious illness and even death. The poisonous substances used are usually sleeping tablets or pain-killing medicines. Gas poisoning is now rare but intentional poisoning with garden and domestic agents is increasing. Although there are two possible motives for taking an overdose,-a genuine wish to die or a rather desperate way of asking for help -it must always be assumed that the victim intended to kill himself. First aid care should involve treatment of the poisoning and constant supervision of the victim until expert medical help is available.

The recovery position

The unconscious patient should be placed in this position provided that his heart is beating at a reasonable rate and his breathing is adequate. Place the poisoned person in a semi prone position with his head down. This will ensure that the tongue falls forward leaving the airways open. If the victim is sick, the vomit will come out of the mouth and not choke the lungs.

Drug addiction

Addiction to dangerous drugs is a growing problem among young people and school children. No-one can experiment with these drugs without running the risk of being permanently trapped. The common addictive drugs can be divided into three types.

The addict may be recognised by his strange behaviour and sometimes by needle-marks and skin infections where drugs have been injected. Drug addiction can kill, or ruin the lives of both the addict and his family. The best cure is prevnetion but if a person is already 'hooked' on drugs, early treatment may help him overcome his addiction. Persuade any addict you know to see his doctor. Do not allow him to keep his awful secret - it could kill him.

Effects of alcohol

Small quantities of alcohol can produce a pleasant state of mind, large quantities dull the brain, impair breathing and may eventually cause death. The drunk is in danger in several ways: he may have an accident, be sick and fill his lungs with vomit, or develop cold exhaustion. Keep him warm and stop him injuring himself. If he is paralytic, place him in the recovery position and get medical help.

Do's

- Check level of consciousness, pulse and breathing regularly and record your results
- Look for evidence of the type of poison taken and see if any note of explanation has been left by the victim
- Get medical help as soon as possible

Don'ts

- Do not give an unconscious victim anything to drink
- Do not make an unconscious victim vomit.
- Do not induce vomiting if the poison is corrosive.

Gas poisoning

The commonest poisonous gas in the home is carbon monoxide. This is present in coal gas but not in North Sea or natural gas. It is also found in exhausts from petrol engines. The victim of carbon monoxide poisoning will be cherry red in colour and will breathe with difficulty. The colour is caused by the carbon monoxide combining with the blood pigment haemoglobin.

You should get to the victim without gassing yourself. Put a cloth over your mouth and quickly approach the victim. Immediately pull the victim into fresh air and start mouth to mouth resuscitation if the victim is either fighting for his breath or has stopped breathing. Check pulse and state of consciousness regularly.

Wasp and bee stings

Remove the sting from the bite with a pair of tweezers. Rinse the wound with a solution of bicarbonate of soda. A soothing lotion such as calamine can be applied. If there is much swelling apply an ice pack. Stings inside the mouth may be dangerous as swelling can interfere with breathing. In this case wash the mouth out with sodium bicarbonate and suck on ice.

Dog, rodent and human bites, treat as simple dirty wounds.

Jelly Fish

These animals produce itchy nettle-rash like stings and can be treated with calamine lotion.

Snake bites

The victim should be made to lie absolutely still and a tourniquet should be placed above the bite. Suck out the poison and go for medical aid. The poisoned person should on no account be given alcohol or any other stimulant.

Poisons in the home and garden

Many tablets found in the home can be very dangerous. Aspirins, paracetamol and iron pills, for example, are all useful medicines but can be poisonous if too many are taken. Coloured tablets are often mistaken for sweets and eaten by unsuspecting children. Keep all medicines in a locked cabinet out of the reach of young children. There are thousands of common household products which can kill if taken by mouth. Oven cleaners, antiseptics cosmetics, and lavatory cleaners are just a few examples. Unfortunately, not all poisons are clearly marked with a poison label or kept in a standard 'poison bottle' with ribbed sides like the one opposite. If any of these are taken the doctor should be called immediately.

Dangerous plants

Another common source of poisons is the garden. The three poisonous plants illustrated below are just a few of the many attractive plants and berries to be found in your own back yard which can kill. If such berries or leaves are eaten, the victim should be encouraged to vomit. Recently weed killers such as paraquat and D.D.T. have been responsible for poisonings. These are dangerous substances. Never store them in lemonade bottles etc. where they might be found by children.

•

Fracture

When a bone breaks, movement and the form of the body is altered and takes on an abnormal shape at the point of the break. A bone which is broken is said to be fractured or cracked. There are different types of fractures and these are listed below. The names are unimportant in themselves but they do serve as a guide to the damage which may be caused by a particular fracture. Any fracture may be described by several of these terms. For example; a break may be a closed, simple fracture or an open, complicated fracture.

Simple fracture: when a bone breaks cleanly in two (like a piece of chalk when dropped on the floor), the fracture is called a simple fracture. Fractures in adults are usually of this kind.

Green stick fracture: a bone which breaks on one side only is said to be a green stick fracture. This is similar to a break in a green piece of wood where the bark tends to hold the ends together.

Complicated and compound fractures: a fracture is termed complicated when the broken ends of the bone tear into other parts of the body such as blood vessels or nerves. Fractures are compound when there is more than one break in the same bone.

Open and closed fractures: when the broken ends of bone puncture the skin and are exposed the fracture is known as "open". If the skin is undamaged then the fracture is said to be "closed".

What does a fracture look like?

The identifying signs of a fracture may be remembered by the word PULSE:

Pain
Unusual shape
Loss of use
Swelling and tenderness
Extra movement
Fractured arm

Treatment

A fracture heals when the broken ends manufacture new bone to cement the break. In order for this process to be effective the bone ends must be held together for a period of time, from a few weeks to months, depending on the site and type of break, and the age and condition of the victim. This is best done by putting a plaster cast around the limb or screwing the bones together with a metal plate. The First-Aider should immobilize the limb to prevent the broken ends from causing pain or further damage. To do this, the joints above and below the break must be prevented from moving. (For example, if the bones of the lower leg are broken the knee and ankle must be immobilized.) In this way, the muscles attached to the broken bone will not be able to shorten and pull the ends apart.

Head Injury

A bang in the head may cause various injuries:

Brain concussion: This occurs when the brain vibrates or shakes within the skull. It temporarily interferes with brain activity and often causes loss of memory and coma. Breathing is shallow and shock may develop. If the victim falls into coma he should be placed in the recovery position and an ambulance called. If the victim regains consciousness, he should be told to seek medical help in case brain compression develops.

Brain compression: This can be caused by a depressed (sunk in) fracture of the skull pressing on the brain or by a blood clot between the skull and the brain. A blood clot can take some time to develop and the first signs of brain compression.may not appear immediately. A person suffering from brain compression usually breathes with difficulty and is flushed in the face. The part of the brain which is compressed does not function properly and part of the body becomes numb and/or paralysed. The victim will become unconscious and should be placed in the recovery position. Send for medical help immediately.

Diabetes

In most people the concentration of sugar in the blood is regulated by a chemical substance called insulin. Diabetics have insufficient insulin to prevent a build up of sugar, and if it becomes too high they will lose consciousness. This condition is called diabetic coma (hyperglycaemia). It is treated by a doctor with insulin injections. If the dose of insulin is too high or if no sugar is eaten, the blood sugar becomes low and the diabetic loses consciousness. This is called insulin coma (hypoglycaemia).

Diabetic coma : This condition occurs only among badly controlled diabetics and first -aiders are not likely to meet it often. It comes on slowly over several days and the diabetic becomes very ill. He often has a smell of nail varnish or pear drops or over-ripe apples on his breath (acetone). There is little that you can do for the victim. Put him in the recovery position and call medical help.

Insulin coma: This type of coma comes on quickly-usually just before a meal-and it is the diabetic problem which first-aiders are more likely to have to deal with. The victim is often angry and difficult to talk to. He may appear to be drunk but there will be no smell of alcohol. Treat this insulin reaction with two tablespoons of sugar in water. You will probably find sugar in his pocket or bag. If he is not given sugar immediately he will quickly become unconscious (insulin coma). In this case place the victim in the recovery position and call a doctor or ambulance. While waiting for the ambulance or doctor put a sugar lump or teaspoonful of sugar in the mouth. A little of this sugar will get into the blood and help the victim. Of course no attempt should be made to make an unconscious victim swallow sugar.

When in doubt: If you are not certain which type of illness the diabetic is suffering from, treat as insulin reaction. Give sugar if the victim is not unconscious.

●

Epilepsy

The brain cells work by a form of biological electricity. Occasionally this electrical system goes wrong and everything discharges at once. This produces an epileptic attack or 'fit'. There are two main types of epileptic fit-major and minor (grand mal and petit mal).

Minor epilepsy (Petit Mal): This usually occurs in children and is nothing more than a short loss of consciousness. It is often so brief that the child looks simply dazed or distant and may not even fall over. There can be many such fits during the day and children get so used to this, they carry on as though nothing has happened.

Major epilepsy (Grand Mal): This is a much more serious condition and takes place in the following order:

Aura: A short warning that a fit is about to happen. It lasts a few seconds or may not occur at all. There is often no time to do anything about it.

Rigid stage: The victim tightens all his muscles and falls to the ground.. He may cry out as all the air is forced from his lungs and he may pass water or open his bowels. He does not breathe and may go blue in the face. This stage lasts only about half a minute so it is not necessary to start mouth to mouth resuscitation. In any case the muscles are so tight that it is impossible to blow air into the lungs.

Shaking stage : This is known as the convulsion. The victim shakes violently. Even the jaw vibrates and the victim may hurt his tongue. After several minutes this stops.

Coma stage: After the convulsion, the epileptic often stays quietly unconscious for about half an hour. During this time he may vomit or obstruct his breathing.

What to do?

Try to prevent injury when the victim falls.

Stop the victim biting his tongue during the shaking stage. This is best done by putting a knotted handkerchief or other soft material between the teeth. But be careful that you are not bitten.

Put the epileptic victim in the recovery position during the coma stage. Make sure the airways remain clear.

If the victim recovers soon (within 15 to 20 minutes) do not call an ambulance. There is nothing more annoying to an epileptic victim than to be taken to a hospital every time he has a fit.

Hysterical reactions

These are caused by an emotional condition which the victim does not understand. The reaction may vary from a temper tantrum to a state which looks like epilepsy. Such fits are dramatic and almost always occur in public. Treat the victim with kindness. Gentle and firm reassurance may be sufficient but if the victim seems unconscious place in the recovery position.

Stroke (Apoplexy)

The brain is supplied with blood by a system of blood vessels which after a .certain point do not connect with each other. If one of these blood vessels bursts or is blocked, then the part of the brain which it supplies will not receive sufficient blood and will stop working. This usually happens in older people.

The right side of the brain controls the left side of the body, and vice versa. If the left side of the brain is short of blood then the right side or part of the right side will not work correctly. It may become numb or paralysed or both. If the area of the brain is large or if certain regions of it are affected, then the victim will become unconscious. There is very little that the First-Aider can do in this situation. Place the victim in the recovery position and call medical help as soon as possible.

First Aid at an Emergency

Working to a clear plan during an emergency will help to ensure that you are effectively prioritising the many demands upon your attention.

Do not allow yourself to become distracted by non-vital activities. Always bear in mind the main steps of emergency action – Assess, Make Safe, Give Emergency Aid, and Get Help.

- Control your feelings. Take a moment to think.
- Do not place yourself in danger.
- Use your common-sense.
- Do not attempt too much alone.
- Be aware of potential dangers such as gas or petrol: use your eyes, ears, and nose to look for clues, for example the hiss of gas or smell of petrol.

Assess the Situation

Your approach should be brisk, but calm and controlled, so that you can quickly take in as much information as possible. Your priorities are to identify any risks to yourself, to the casualty, and to any bystanders, then to assess the resources available to you and the kind of help you may need. State that you have first aid skills when offering your help. If there are no doctors, nurses, or more experienced people present, calmly take charge. First ask yourself these questions:

- is there any continuing danger?
- is anyone's life in immediate danger?
- are there bystanders who can help?
- do I need specialist help?

Make the Area Safe

The conditions that caused the accident may still be presenting further danger. Remember that you must put your own safety first. You cannot help others if you become a casualty yourself.

Often, very simple measures, such as turning off an electric switch, are enough to make the area safe. Sometimes more complicated procedures are required. Never put yourself and the casualty at further risk by attempting to do too much; be aware of your limitations.

Dealing with ongoing danger

If you cannot eliminate a life-threatening hazard, you must try to put some distance between it and the casualty, by attempting to remove the danger from the casualty if possible. As a last resort, remove the casualty from the danger. In many situations, you will need specialist help and equipment.

Give Emergency Aid

Once it is safe, quickly make an initial assessment of each casualty following the ABC of resuscitation. So that any casualty needing emergency first aid is treated immediately.

Establish whether each casualty:

- is conscious:
- has an open airway;
- is breathing
- has a pulse.

Your findings dictate, your priorities and when and how much help is needed.

Get Help

You may be faced with a number of tasks to maintain safety, to telephone for help, and to start first aid. Other people can be asked to:

- make the area safe;
- telephone for assistance;

- fetch first-aid equipment; control traffic and onlookers; control bleeding or support a limb;
- maintain the casualty's privacy; transport the casualty to a safe place

The control of onlookers

The reaction of bystanders may cause you concern or even anger. Most of them will have no first-aid training and that could make them feel helpless or frightened. If they have witnessed or been involved in the incident, they too may be injured without realising it, and will certainly be distressed. If you need to ask a bystander to help, do so in a firm, but gentle manner.

Telephoning for Help

You can summon help by telephone, from a number of sources.

Emergency services: police, fire, and ambulance services; mine, mountain, cave and fell rescue.

- Utilities: gas, electricity, and water.
- Health services: doctor, dentist, nurse or midwife.

If you have to leave a casualty alone, minimise risk to him or her by taking any vital action first. Make your call short but accurate.

Finding a Telephone

Emergency calls are free, and can be made on any telephone, including most mobile and car phones. On motorways, emergency telephones can be found every mile; marker posts between them indicate the nearest box. These telephones simply need to be picked up to be answered.

Most large companies have special arrangements for calling for assistance. Make sure that you are familiar with them. If you ask someone else to make the call, ask them to come, back and confirm that help is on the way.

Making the Call

On dialling emergency, you will be asked which service you require, and will be put through to the appropriate control officer. Whenever there are casualties involved, ask for the ambulance service; the control officer can, if necessary, pass on messages to other emergency services.

When you get through to the control officer, give clear details of the accident or emergency. If you are not sure of your precise location, do not panic – your call can be traced to any call box or motorway telephone. Do not put the telephone down until the control officer clears the line.

You may be required to stay by the telephone to "lead in" the emergency services. If you delegate this task, make sure that the person understands its importance and reports back to you.

Calling the Emergency Services

State your name clearly and that you are acting in your capacity as a First Aider.

The following details are essential

- Your telephone number.
- The exact location of the incident; a road name or number, if possible, and any junctions or other landmarks.
- The type and gravity of the incident, for example, "Traffic accident, two cars, road blocked, three people are trapped"
- The number, sex, and approximate ages of the casualties, and anything you know about their condition, for example, "Man, early fifties, suspected heart attack, cardiac arrest".
- Details of any hazards such as gas, hazardous substances, power-line damage, or relevant weather conditions, for example fog or ice.

Multiple Casualties

In situations such as major traffic accidents, you may find yoursell in the difficult position of having to deal with several casualties at the same time. You may be on your own, working with other first aiders, or with professionals. A methodical and calm approach will be crucial in the initial chaos. Always follow the ABC of resuscitation in order to establish treatment priority, and attend first to any unconscious casualty. Remember, you can only do your best in these circumstances.

Major Incidents

Major incidents involving a large number of casualties may place overwhelming demands on rescuers. The first task is to ensure that the emergency services are contacted immediately and given accurate information about the incident. The next priority is to assess the scene, and providing it is safe to do so, to start giving emergency first aid.

If other First Aiders come forward, give them as much information as possible. The most senior First Aider present should take charge of the team. When the emergency services arrive, the senior officer will take absolute control.

The role of the First Aider

At major public events, especially when there is a doctor on your team, you constitute the on-site medical team untill hospital and other services arrive. When they do arrive, your role will diminish.

At any major incident, you must leave the scene if asked to do so by a member of the emergency services. However, you may be asked to help the medical teams by performing simple tasks, for example holding drips or supporting limbs. Always do as you are asked; your help will be greatly appreciated.

When a major accident occurs, the police will establish rendezvous points and nominate officers for all rescuers to report to. It is vital not to disturb any evidence on site, especially following fatal accidents, as there may be a legal inquiry.

How you can help?

Identify the serious casualties and mark them for immediate treatment. Move casualties with minor injuries quickly from the site to allow access to serious cases; minor injuries can be treated when time allows. This process is called triage.

- Casualties who are obviously dead should be left, so that help can be given to those who need it.
- All those involved should be logged, and casualties labelled, so that accurate records can be made and maintained.
- Workers or residents at or near the site of a disaster should be alerted to security risks and any further hazards.

Road Accidents

Road accidents range from a fall from a bicycle to a major incident with many casualties. Often, the accident site will present serious risks to safety, largely because of passing traffic. It is essential to make the area safe - to protect yourself, the casualty, and other road users.

Make the Accident Site Safe

First ensure your own safety; and do not do anything that might create danger.

- Park safely; well clear of the accident site. Set your hazard lights flashing.
- Do not run across a busy motorway
- At night, wear or carry something light or reflective, and use a torch. Then take these general precautions.
- Send bystanders to warn other drivers.

- Set up warning triangles or lights 200 metres (250 yards) in each direction. Switch off the ignition of any damaged vehicle and, if you can, disconnect the battery. Switch off the fuel supply on diesel vehicles and motorcycles.

Stabilise vehicles

If a vehicle is upright, apply the hand-brake and put it in gear, or put blocks at the wheels. If a vehicle is on its side, do not right it, but try to prevent it from rolling over. Look out for physical dangers. Is anyone, smoking? Are there goods vehicles displaying Hazchem symbols? Are there damaged power lines or spill fuel? If you see a radiation hazard sign, make sure that you alert the police immediately.

Hazardous Substances

Accidents may be complicated by the spillage of dangerous substances or the escape of toxic vapours. Never make a rescue attempt unless you are sure that you will not come, into contact with a dangerous substance. Keep bystanders away from the scene, bearing in mind that poisonous fumes may be released and travel some distance. Stand upwind of the accident to ensure that any fumes are blown away from you.

Hazchem symbols

A Hazchem placard on a vehicle warns that it is carrying a hazardous substance. In doubt about your safety or the meaning of the sign, keep your distance, especially if there is any spillage, or if you see the letter "E". The information is coded and will be understood by that emergency services, so make a note of it and pass it on when telephoning for help.

Check the Casualties

Quickly assess all casualties, while moving them. Search the area thoroughly, so that if they are in danger or you need not overlook a casualty who may have so to apply life-saving treatment. Deal been thrown clear in the accident or have with life-threatening conditions first, wandered away while confused.

For a Casualty Trapped under a Vehicle

1. Mark the exact position of the vehicle and the casualty first. The police will need this information.
2. Try to find help to lift or move the vehicle and, only if it is absolutely necessary, drag the casualty clear.

For an Unconscious Casuality

1. Assume there is a neck injury until proved otherwise. Support the head and neck with your hands, so that the casualty can breathe freely. Apply a collar, if possible.
   DO NOT move the casulaty unless it is absolutely necessary.
2. Treat any life-threatening injuries if possible. Monitor and record breathing, pulse, and level of response every ten minutes.

If it is essential to move the casuality you will need three people to help you: one to support the shoulders and chest, one for the hips and abdomen, and one for the legs. Support the casualty's head continuously and direct all movements.

●

Fire Injuries

Rapid, clear thinking at a fire is vital. Fire spreads very quickly, so warn any people at risk, and alert the emergency services immediately. Panic also spreads quickly so you must calm anyone who is likely to increase alarm.

If leaving a burning building, try to help everyone out of the building without putting yourself at risk. Shut all doors behind you. Look for fire exits and assembly points. You should know, the evacuation procedure, at your workplace. If visiting business premises, follow instructions given by staff.

If arriving at a fire or burns incident, STOP, OBSERVE, THINK, and DO NOT RUSH IN. There may be flammable or explosive substances, such as gas, or toxic fumes or a risk of electrocution. A minor fire can escalate in minutes to a serious blaze. If there is a risk to you, wait for the emergency services.

Leaving a Burning Building

1. Activate the first fire alarm you see.
2. Close each door behind you as you go.
3. Do not run, but walk quickly and calmly.

Dealing with a Fire

A fire needs three components to start and maintain it: ignition (an electric spark or naked flame); a source of fuel (petrol, wood or fabric); and oxygen (air). Remove any one of these to break this "triangle of fire". For example:

- switch off a car's ignition or pull the fuel cut-off on large diesel vehicles;

- remove from the path of a fire any combustible materials, such as curtains or cardboard, that may fuel the flames;
- shut a door on fire to cut off its oxygen supply; smother flames with a smoke blanket or other impervious substance.

Clothing on Fire

Always follow the same procedure for a casualty with burning clothing: STOP, DROP, AND ROLL, if possible, wrap the casualty before rolling them.

What you can do?

- STOP the casualty from panicking or running around or outside; any movement or breeze will fan the flames.
- DROP the casualty to the ground.
- If possible, WRAP the casualty tightly in a coat, curtain, blanket (not the nylon or cellular type), rug or other heavy fabric. The best fabric for this is wool.
- ROLL the casualty along the ground until the flames have been smothered.

If water or another non-flammable liquid is readily available, lay the casualty down with burning side uppermost, and extinguish the flames by dousing him in plenty of the liquid.

If your own clothes catch fire and help is not available, extinguish the flames by wrapping yourself up lightly in suitable material, and rolling along the ground.

Smoke and Fumes

Any fire in a confined space creates a highly dangerous atmosphere that is low in oxygen and may be contaminated by carbon monoxide and toxic fumes. Never enter a burning or fume-filled building, or open a door leading to a fire. Leave it to the emergency services.

What you can do?

- If trapped in a burning building, go into a room with a window and shut the door. If you must pass through a smoke-filled room, keep low down: the air at floor level is the clearest.

If you have to escape through a window, go out feet first and lower yourself to the full length of your arms before dropping to the ground.

•

Electrical Injuries

When a person is electrocuted, the passage of electrical current through the body may stun the casualty causing breathing and even the heart to stop. The current may cause burns both where it enters the body and where it leaves the body to go to "earth". Alternating current also causes muscle spasms that often prevent the casualty from letting go of an electric cable, so the casualty may still be 'live' when you come on the scene.

Lighting

A natural burst of electricity discharged from the atmosphere, lightning forms an intense trail of light and heat that seeks contact with the ground through the nearest tall feature in the landscape, and, possibly, anyone standing by it. A lightning strike may set clothing on fire and knock the casualty clown. Occasionally, it may cause instant death. Clear everyone from the site of a lightning strike as soon as possible.

Hight-voltage Current

Contact with high-voltage current, found in power lines and overhead high-tension (HT) cables, is usually immediately fatal. Severe burns always result. The sudden muscular spasm produced by the shock may propel the casualty some distance, causing injuries such as fractures High-voltage electricity may jump (arc) up to 18 metres (20 yards). Materials such as dry wood or clothing will not protect you. The power must be cut out and isolated before you approach the casualty. This is crucial where railway overhead power lines are damaged.

Action

DO NOT approach the casualty until you are officially told that the power has been cut off and, if necessary isolated. Maintain a safe distance of 18 metres (20 yards) or more and keep any bystanders away.

1. DIAL 100 FOR THE EMERGENCY SERVICES
2. The casualty will probably be unconscious; once it is safe to do so, open the airway, check breathing and pulse, and be ready to resuscitate if necessary. Place him in the recovery position.
3. Treat any burns and associated injuries.
4. Take steps to minimise the effects of shock

Low-Voltage Current

Domestic current, as used in homes, offices, workshops, and shops, can cause serious injury, and even death. Many injuries result from faulty switches, frayed ilex, or defects within an appliance itself. Young children are especially at risk.

You must be aware of the hazards of water which is a dangerously efficient conductor of electricity. Handling an otherwise safe appliance with wet hands or when standing on a wet floor, greatly increases the risk of a shock.

Action

DO NOT touch the casualty if he is in contact with the electrical current; he will be 'live' and you risk electrocution.

DO NOT use anything metallic to push away the electrical source.

Break the contact by switching off the current, at the mains or meter point if it can be reached easily. Otherwise, remove the plug or wrench the cable free.

If you are unable to reach the cable, socket, or mains, follow this procedure: Stand on dry insulating material such as a wooden box, a rubber or plastic mat, a telephone directory or a thick pile of newspaper. Push the casualty's limbs away from the source with a broom, wooden chair or stool, or push the source away from the casualty, whichever is easier.

- Without touching the casualty, loop rope around his feet or under the arms and pull him away from the source.
- If absolutely necessary, pull the casualty free by pulling at his loose, dry clothing. Do this only as a last resort.
- If the casualty is unconscious, open the airway, check breathing and pulse, and be ready to resuscitate if necessary. Place him in the recovery position. Cool any burns with cold water.
- DIAL EMERGENCY FOR AN AMBULANCE.

  IF the casualty seems to be unharmed, he should be advised to rest. Observe him closely and, if in doubt, call a doctor.

If the Heart stops

Apply the ABC of resuscitation until a normal heartbeat returns or specific medical treatment is given. If trained, a blow with the heel of a hand on the centre of the chest may help, but this should be tried only twice.

Rescue from Drowning

Open water in and around Britain is cold, even in summer. Temperatures in the sea range from 5°C (41°F) to 15°C (59°F); inland waters may be even colder. The cold increases the dangers to both the casualty and rescuer, as it may cause:

- uncontrollable gasping on entering the water, with the consequent risk of water inhalation;
- a sudden rise in blood pressure, which can precipitate a heart attack;
- sudden inability to swim – hypothermia – if immersion i n the water is prolonged or the casualty is exposed to the wind.

Action

YOUR AIMS ARE:

- To get the casualty on 10 dry land with minimum danger to yourself.
- To treat the casualty for drowning and hypothermia, if necessary
- To arrange removal to hospital.

1. Choose the safest way to rescue the casualty Remember to REACH AND THROW. Don't go into the water. Stay on land and reach out with your hand, a stick or branch, or throw a rope or a float.

- If you are a trained life-saver, or if the casualty is unconscious, you may have to swim to the casualty and tow him to dry land. It is safer to wade than to swim.

  DO NOT enter the water yourself unless it is absolutely necessary.

IF the casualty is unconscious, carry her with her head lower than her chest once she is clear of the water, to minimise risk of vomiting.

2. Shield the casualty from the wind if possible, to prevent the body from being chilled any further (this is known as the "wind chill" factor).
3. Treat the casualty for drowning and the effects of severe cold.
4. Arrange to take or send the casualty to hospital, even if he or she seems to have recovered well or, if necessary.

●

Stress – How to Overcome?

Even the most experienced First Aider in an emergency situation can be upsetting. It is natural to feel stressed. Whenever you are called upon to administer first aid, and to be very emotional once you have finished treating the casualty.

It is likely that the incident will affect you afterwards, so it is important to face up to how you feel and what has happened. In extreme cases, you may experience the more serious condition, Post-traumatic Stress Disorder.

Coping during an Emergency

Many First Aiders worry that they might not be able to cope in a real-life situation. Infact, your body has a natural mechanism that prompts you to act quickly in an emergency. In the "fight or flight" response (see right), your body is prepared for physical exertion. So the stress you will feel is your body's way of getting you through a difficult situation.

Calming down

Although the "fight or flight" response is beneficial, sometimes too a great rush of adrenaline may affect your ability to cope. Lying slow, deep breaths will help you calm down, leaving you better able to remember your first-aid procedures.

"Fight or Flight" Response

When faced with any stressful situation, the body will automatically respond by releasing the hormones, adrenaline, noradrenaline, and cortisol, which prepare the body to "fight or Hight". This response occurs in all animals as a reaction to a threatening or stressful situation, but in the human body the signs include:

- a pounding heart;
- deep, fast breathing;
- pupils widening to let in more light;
- increased sweating;
- alertness of mind;
- greater blood flow to the muscles;
- a rise in blood sugar level for energy.

Feelings after the Incident

After you have treated the casualty, depending on the type of incidence and the outcome, you might experience:

Satisfaction and pleasure – it is nature to feel good about yourself. If the treatment has gone well;

Confusion and doubt – you might question your actions and feel you could have done more, especially if the outcome is unclear;

Anger and sadness – being upset is normal, especially in major incidents;

Releasing these feelings at the time will help you get over the event more quickly.

Delayed Reaction

Involvement in an incident can lead to stress once you have returned to your normal, everyday environment. The extent of the effect may depend on the level of your first-aid experience and the type of incident, and it is important to recognise the signs and deal with your feelings as soon as possible.

Symptoms and signs

Stress can lead to interference with a person's physical and mental well-being, and some people are more susceptible to it than others. It is quite normal to suffer from some stress after a traumatic event. Stress can manifest itself in very many different ways, but these symptoms should pass in time.

Recognition there may be:

- Tremor of the hands and stomach.
- Excessive sweating. Flashbacks of the incident.
- Nightmares or disturbed sleep.
- Tearfulness.
- Tension and irritability
- A feeling of withdrawal and isolation.

Dealing with Stress

If you experience stress after an incident, do not think that you are weak or overreacting. It is important that you do not bottle up your feelings as this will cause you more stress. Your feelings can also be relieved by exercise or relaxation techniques, such as meditation or yoga. In fact, doing any activity that you enjoy is a good way to relax and may help to relieve tension.

Talking to a friend

Face up to what has happened by confiding in a friend or a relative. Ideally, speak to someone who also attended the incident: you may find! They have the same feelings as yours.

Dealing with stress alone

Try writing down your feelings and what happened, including all the positive actions you took. You can then use this as a talking point.

Post-Traumatic Stress Disorder (PTSD)

If you have witnessed or experienced a serious threat to life or physical well-being, and suffer all of the following symptoms, you may have Post-traumatic Stress Disorder: relieving the event in some way;

- persistent avoidance of situations, people or situations associated with the event;
- persistent hyperactivity;
- symptoms that appear more than 30 days after the event, and last for a minimum of a month.

The condition can be made worse by reminders of the event, and it is important to see a doctor or counsellor for help.

The Practice of First Aid

In most situations that require first aid, there will be no life-threatening danger. You will simply be assisting a conscious casualty; whose recovery from some minor injury or illness is not in doubt. In all cases, your aim is to work to a plan and discover what is wrong with the casualty, and to give prompt, correct treatment in a methodical way.

Assessing the situation

Before tending to a casualty, however, you must survey the whole scene. Your first responsibility is to make sure that the area is safe. Often hazards such as passing traffic can be dealt with simply, but where the danger is too great or too imminent, you may need to move the casualty even at the risk of aggravating the injury. Do this only if it is safe to approach the casualty: you cannot help others if you also become a casualty. Only when the casualty is safe can you begin to treat the illness or injury.

The first aider should:

- Preserve life
- Pay strict attention to safety
- Follow the ABC of resuscitation
- Control any major bleeding
- Limit worsening of the condition
- Make a diagnosis of the injury or illness, if possible, by means of a thorough examination.
- Give priority to seriously injured casualties.

- Treat multiple injuries in order of priority dealing with life-threatening conditions first. Consider the possibility of "hidden" secondary conditions.
- Promote the casualty's recovery.
- Relieve any discomfort, pain or anxiety. Arrange for appropriate medical attention.

How People React and How to Help

When involved in a serious accident people react in different ways. They get themselves into a "state".

Step One	See and recognise obvious injuries.
Step Two	Check pulse, breathing, level of consciousness, signs of bleeding.
Step Three	Start at the head and work down to the toes. Look for bleeding, tenderness or signs. Take each limb in turn and of a fracture, then the chest and abdomen. If the victim is conscious talk to him as you do this.
Step Four	Ask if the casualty is being seen by the doctor or treated for any disease. If the casualty is unconscious make a search for: Medic-alert Information Diabetic cards etc. The name and address of the victim.
Step Five	Always look for signs of shock.
Step Six	Check and check again pulse breathing, level of consciousness. Is bleeding controlled?

State of fear: Fear or anxiety is probably the most common reaction. It can be recognised by trembling, gooseflesh, a rapid heart beat and restlessness. It must be treated by calming the victim, talking gently and reassuringly. A warm blanket, a friendly face and as much good news as possible will provide much comfort.

State of grief: Another common reaction is sudden sadness or grief. In this situation the victim usually sobs or remains quiet and withdrawn. This responds to encouraging the victim to talk to you. Stay with him, listen to him, say as little as possible and do not pester him with needless questions.

State of excitement: When the victim gabbles uncontrollably and overreacts to every stimulus he must be sheltered from the chaos and activity at the scene of the accident. Quiet, rest and firm instructions are necessary.

State of confusion: Any sudden event such as an accident especially after an injury to the head may make the casualty confused. This is easily recognised when the victim asks the same question time and again, loses his grasp of the situation, or becomes disorientated. Such an injury needs a quiet situation and the constant reassuring presence of the same person.

State of forgetfulness: If the victim has forgotten how he became injured, what happened before or after the accident or even what his name and address is, you should make a special note of this. It probably indicates concussion and he should certainly see a doctor.

Redirect traffic: Do not rush on to the road without first making sure that it is safe to cross. Switch off the car's engine and disconnect the battery if possible. Set reflective triangles or other warning devices some 50 metres on both sides of the accident. If there is fast moving traffic on the road the warning triangles should be moved even further from the crash.

Send for help

Check the victim: If he is not breathing start immediate mouth-to-mouth resuscitation: if the heart has stopped initiate external cardiac compression.

Do not move the victim: Unless the car is on fire, he is in danger of being hit by oncoming traffic, or his breathing or heart has stopped, the victim should not be disturbed.

Do not smoke: Petrol may have spilled on the roadway and the cigarette could cause a fire or explosion.

Do not give alcohol: This would not help the victim medically and the police might think he had been drinking while driving.

Fire

A fire extinguisher, blanket or earth may be used to fight a fire, but an explosion may occur. If there is a fire move yourself and the victim away immediately. Never use water as this may spread the flames.

Trapped victim

Check his respiration and pulse. If he is not breathing, start immediate mouth to mouth resuscitation. If the heart has stopped do not waste a lot of time trying to free him from the wreck but begin external cardiac compression. Delay will most certainly result in the victim's death. It may be difficult to perform the external cardiac compression properly, but do the best you can.

Spinal injury

- Is the victim complaining of a pain in the back?
- Does he have difficulty in moving his fingers or toes?
- Has any part of his body become numb?

If so, it is likely that there has been an injury to the spine. A common site of such injuries at a road accident is in the neck. Roll up a newspaper and secure it round the neck with string to reduce the possibility of further injury. Do not move the victim unless it is absolutely necessary to do so, as this could cause further injury which could lead to paralysis.

REMEDIES FOR BRUISES

Remedies	Specific Indications	Worse From	Better From
Arnica	Common bruises, Injuries from blow or fall, Shock	Least touch, Rest	Lying down, Head low
Hypericum (Internally or lotion)	Crushing injuries to nerves, Nerve injury to: "Crazybones", Fingertips, Nailbeds, Palms, Soles of feet, Tailbones, Toes, Puncture wounds	Cold, Touch	
Ledum (Internally or lotion)	Bruises: Cold and numb bruised parts, Long-lasting black eye, Splinter under nail, Bruised nerves, Puncture wounds	Warmth	Bathing in cold water
Ruta	Injuries of: Bones, Periosteum, Bone covering, Shins, Soft tissue, Prolapsed, Protruding rectum, Wrist and ankle sprains	Lying down, Cold, Wet weather	

REMEDIES FOR SPRAINS

Remedies	General Indications	First-Aid Measures
Arnica (Internally or Lotion)	Shock of injury, Bleeding in tissues	Massage injured area gently with *Arnica* oil or lotion, but only on unbroken skin. Elvate injured part. During the first 24 hours, apply ice bag or cold compress to painful area to reduce swelling and pain; apply heat after that. Warp injured area with elastic bandage for support.
Bryonia	Injured joint swollen, Distended, Painful Worse on movement®	
Ledium	Injured joint cold and numb, Much swelling	
Rhus toxicodendron	After *Arnica* Hot, swollen, painful joint, Creaky on first movement; better when limbered up.	
Ruta graveolens	Torn and wrenched tendons or ligaments Bruised periosteum (bone covering), Worse in cold wet weather. After *Arnica* and *Ruta*..	
Symphytum (Internally and lotion)	If necessary, Injury to sinews, tendons and the bone . covering	
Arunica	Sore, Bruised feeling, Strained back muscles, Sore muscles	Elevate the injured part. Apply cold packs during the first 24 hours; heat after that. Wrap loosely with elastic bandage to support injured area.
Rhus toxica- dendraom	Sore muscles, Torn ligaments and tendons Bruised periosteum (bone covering). Worse on first movement batter after limbered up.	

REMEDIES FOR WOUNDS

Remedies	General Indications and Benefits	Worse From	Better From
Arnica	Shock of injury, Speeds healing, Jagged wounds (internal use only)	Light touch, Heat, Rest	Head low
Calendula	Cleanses and speeds healing of: Abrasions (lotion), Scratches (lotion), Superficial wounds (Lotion)		
Hepar Sulphur	Red, Swollen, Painful wounds	Lying on painful side, Slight touch, Slightest draft	Warmth
Hypericum	Relieves nerve pain and pain of jagged wounds, Cleanses and speeds healing of Jagged, irregular cuts (lotion), Lacerations (Lotion), Painful burns (lotion).	Touch, cold	Bending head backward
Ledum	Cleanses puncture wounds (lotion)	Night, Heat of the bed, Warm applications	Cold applications

INSECT BITES AND STINGS

Remedies	General Indications	Worse From	Better From
Apis Bee for Hornet and Wasp Stings	Burning, Stinging pains, Rapid rosy swelling, not bright red, Puffiness rather than hard swelling	Heat, Hot applications	
Arnica (Tincture) Bee for Hornet and Wasp Stings	Applied directly to the sting, relieves pain at once	Least touch, Rest	Lying down with head low
Calendula (Tincture) Bee for Hornet and Wasp Stings	Relieves pain and swelling when applied directly to sting		
Cantharis, Bee for Hornet and Wasp Stings	Red and inflamed stings, Burning sensation	Touch	Gentle massage
Carbolicum acidum for Poisonous Spider,	Dusky red face, Pale around mouth and nose, Listless, sluggish Sensitive to odors		

INSECT BITES AND STINGS

Remedies	General Indications	Worse From	Better From
Scorpio and Snake Bites			
Crotalus horridus, Poisonous Spider, Scorpion, and Snake Bites	Rapid, violent onset of symptoms, Much swelling, Discoloration around bite	Jarring	
Echinacea Poisonous Spider, Scorpio and Snake Bites	Red streaks Blood poisoning and infection Sepsis, foul-smelling discharge		
Hypericum (Internally or tincture) for Bee, Hornet, and Wasp Stings	Severe pain shooting upward	Cold, Touch	Bending head backward

INSECT BITES AND STINGS

Remedies	General Indications	Worse From	Better From
Lachesis for Poisonous Spider, Scorpio and Snake Bites	Affected part dusky red or blue, Oozing of dark blood	After sleep	
Ledum (Internally or tincture) for Bee, Hornet, and Wasp Stings	Punctured wounds and stings, Numbness or high sensitiviy or high sensitivity to touch, Pains extend upward, Wounded parts may be cold	Night, Heat of the bed	Cold applications Cold bathing
Oxalicum acidum Poisonous Spider, Scorpion, and Snake Bites	Affected part cold and numb Violent pain Trembling of hands and feet	Slightest touch Thinking about himself	

REMEDIES FOR BURNS

Remedies	Instructions
Arnica	To be given first to prevent shock.
Cantharis	If pain persists after *Arnica,* give 2 tablets every 15 minutes until pain lessens. Repeat *Cantharis* if pain returns.
Causticum	If the pain is accompanied by restlessness and blister formation, give 2 tablets of *Causticum* every 15 minutes until pain lessens.
Aloe Vera	Gel from plant forms a protective covering, relieves pain and promotes healing.
Calendula Lotion	Immerse burned area in cold water with a few drops of *Calendula* succus or tincture. Saturate dressing with *Calendula* lotion to cleanse, relieve pain and heal.
Hypericum Lotion	Immerse burned area in cold *Hypericum* lotion. Dressing should be saturated with *Hypericum* lotion and applied to burned area to prevent serum loss and promote tissue formation.
Urtica urens	Soothing lotion when applied externally, quickly relieves pain and heals. When older burns are characterized by itching and stinging, *Urtica* lotion relieves.

SPORTS INJURIES

Injury	Remedy	First-Aid Measures
Athlete's Foot	*Calendula*	Wash feet thoroughly with water and mild soap (preferably *Calendula* soap). Apply *Calendula* ointment. Expose feet to air. Avoid synthetic or colored hose.
Bleeding from mouth	*Calendula*	Rinse mouth with *Calendula* lotion.
Blisters	*Cantharis*	Clean area, bandage to protect from pressure and dirt.
Raw burning pains; Better from cold applications		
Burning heat	*Urtica*	
Broken Rib Pain	*Bryonia*	Rest in comfortable position. Avoid jarring.
When pain lessens, To promote healing of bone	*Symphytum*	
Bruises (Black eye, face bruise, heel or toe bruise, knee bruise barked skin, strains)	*Arnica*	Cleanse if necessary, Place ice pack over bruise.
Crushed Fingers and Toes	*Hypericum*	Rest and elevate injured part.

SPORTS INJURIES

Injury	Remedy	First-Aid Measures
Cuts and Abrasions General	*Calendula Lotion*	Clean area gently but throughly with mild soap and water, rinse in clear water, then apply *Calendula* lotion. Apply a sterile, nonstick gauze dressing with *Calendula* lotion..
Nerves (toes, fingers etc.)	*Hypericum Lotion*	Follow directions above, but substitue *Hypericum* lotion.
Fractures For shock and pain	*Arnica*	Keep patient warm and treat with *Arnica* to prevent shock. Apply ice to painful area. If victim with broken bone must be moved, improvise a splint to keep bones from moving.
Jock Itch	*Calendula Lotion or Ointment*	Keep groin area clean and dry. Apply *Calendula* lotion or ointment. Use corn starch as dusting powder.
Nosebleed, Profuse bleeding from vigorous nose-blowing	*Phosphores*	Sit quietly with head thrown forward. Pinch nostrils together for 5 to 10 minutes.
Bright red blood; gushing	*Ipecac*	If bleeding continues, pack nostril with plug or sterile gauze. Lie down on your back with head elevated and cold wet cloth across face.
Overexertion Bruised sore feeling. Aching muscles and joints. General fatigue	*Arnica*	Rest followed by gentle exercise to limber up muscles. Warm, relaxing bath.

SPORTS INJURIES

Injury	Remedy	First-Aid Measures
Shin Splints	*Arnica*	Apply ice pack to reduce pain; then heat treatment and gentle massage.
Sore Muscles	*Arnica* (Internally and lotion)	Externally, massage injured area with *Arnica* oil or lotion.
Sprained Ankle or Wrist if better from cold aplications	*Ledum*	Massage injured area gently with *Arnica* oil or lotion, but never on broken skin.
After swelling reduced	*Arnica* (Internally and lotion)	Elevate the injured part; apply cold pack during first 24 hours; heat after that.
After *Arnica*, if necessary	*Ruta graveolens*	Support injured joint with losely wrapped elastic bandage.
If weakness is still present after 2 weeks	*Calcarea carbonica*	Do as above.
Strained Muscles, Tendons, Ligaments	*Rhus toxicodendron*	Elevate the injured part; apply cold pack during first 24 hours, heat after that Wrap injured area with elastic bandage for support.
Sunstroke and Heat Exhaustion, Face hot and flushed, Bursting headache, Waves of throbbing	*Glonine*	Move victim to cool or shady place. Put cold wet cloth on head. When conscious give one teaspoon of salt in a pint of water, encourage victim to drink several glasses.

SPORTS INJURIES

Injury	Remedy	First-Aid Measures
Pupils dilated. Pulse strong, pounding, Skin burning, dry flushed	*Belladonna*	
Nausea, Pallor, Clammy sweat, Prostration Pulse rapid and feeble	*Veratrum album*	
Cramping, in addition to *Veratrum album* symptoms	*Cuprum metallicum*	
Tendonitis (Inflamed tendon) Painful when beginning to move; better after continued motion, Worse in damp weather	*Rhus toxicodendron*	Wrap with elastic bandage to limit motion in painful joint
Lame feeling, Lacks distinct characteristics of *Rhus tox.*	*Ruta* *Ruta*	
Tennis Elbow	*Arnica*	Apply ice and rest the arm for a few days.
Twisted Knee	*Bryonia*	Apply cold pack during first 24 hours, heat after that.
Take on first day		Wrap the injured part to limit motion.
If worse from slightest motion; take on second day		Elevate and rest the injured knee.

REMEDIES FOR EMERGENCIES

Remedy	General Indications	Worse From	Better From
Aconite For every Injury	To diminish inflamation, To relieve pain	Night Warm room	Open air
For Conditions with fever	Sudden onset, Restless, Fearful	Lying on painful side	
Apis mellifica For Breathing difficulty	Allergic shock, Reactions to bee stings, Throat passages closed, Tongue swollen	Heat, Touch, Hot applications Pressure	Motion, Cold bath, Open air
Antimonium tartaricum For Breathing difficulty	Cardiac failure: drowning in own secretions Drowning: cold and blue patient; respiration ratting, Respiratory failures: drowning in own secretion; clammy sweat	Evening Warmth Lying down at night	Sitting erect, Belching, Expectoration
Arnica For Bleeding	Caused by injury	Least touch	Lying down
For Eye injury	Black eye, Injury to socket, Soft tissue surrounding eye	Rest	Head low

REMEDIES FOR EMERGENCIES

Remedy	General Indications	Worse From	Better From
For Shock	From injury		
Arsenicum album For Asthma	Unable to lie down, afraid of suffocation Wheezing respiration, Great debility, Burning in chest Worse from 1 to 2 A.M.	After midnight, Cold	Warmth, Warm drinks Head elevated
For Conditions with fever	Restless, Anxious, Burning pains, Thirsty for frequent small sips		
For Food poisoning	Vomiting and diarrhea		
Belladonna For Conditions with fever	Sudden onset, Violent symptoms, Face flushed, Skin burning to the touch, Restless	Afternoon, Lying down, Touch, Jarring, Noise	Being semierect
For Sunstroke	Pupils dilated, Pulse strong, pounding, Skin burning, dry flushed		
Bryonia For Conditions with	Thirsty for large drinks, Skin pale, Irritable,	Motion, Touch	Rest Quiet

REMEDIES FOR EMERGENCIES

Remedy	General Indications	Worse From	Better From
fever	Desires quiet	Warmth	
Calendula (lotion) For Eye injury	Control of bleeding		
Carbo vegetabilis For Asthma	Onset after long spasmodic coughing spell with gagging and vomiting, Sore raw chest with difficult breathing, especially in evening, Air hunger; must be fanned, Bluish face; cold breath, Symptoms worse after eating or talking	Evening, Open air, Wine Warm, damp weather	Belching Fanning
For Bleeding, External or Internal	Dark blood, steady oozing		
For Collapse	From any cause, Air hunger, Cold breath, Sweat, cold and clammy		
Chamomilla For Fainting	From severe pain	Night, Open air, Heat	Being carried, Warm wet weather

REMEDIES FOR EMERGENCIES

Remedy	General Indications	Worse From	Better From
For Intolerance of pain		Anger	
China For blood loss resulting in:	Air hunger (gasping for breath), Faintness, Ringing in ears, Dimming of vision	Slightest touch, Draft, After eating, Loss of vital fluids	Hard pressure, Open air, Warmth
For After-effects of loss of any vital fluids	With weakness and any of the above		
Coffea For Fainting	From excitement	Excessive emotions Strong odors Noise	Warmth Lying down
For Sleeplessness	From excitement or joy	Open air, Cold	Holding ice in mouth
Cuprum metallicum For Heat exhaustion	Cramping in addition to *Veratrum album* symptoms	Contact Vomiting	Perspiring Drinking cold water
Ferrum phosphoricum	Red cheeks, Gradual onset	Right side, Night 4 to 6 A.M.,	Cold applications

REMEDIES FOR EMERGENCIES

Remedy	General Indications	Worse From	Better From
For Conditions with fever	Soft and rapid pulse	Touch, Jar, Motion	
Gelsemium For Conditions with fever	Aching, Chilly Drooping eyes	Excitement, Damp weather	Open air, Continued motion, Profuse urination
For Influenza	Lethargic	Left side, 6 A.M. to	Brandy
Glonine For Sunstroke	Face hot and flushed, Bursting headache, Waves of throbbing, Skin sweaty	noon Motion, Jarring, Stooping, Lying down	
		Dry, cold weather	Warmth, After eating
Hepar sulphur For Fainting	From slight pain Excessive and long-lasting pain,	Cold, Touch	Damp weather Bending head backward
Hypericum For Eye injury	Pain after removal of foreign object (lotion as an eyewash)		
Ipecacuanha For Asthma	Sudden onset, Wheezing; gasps for air, Must sit up breath, Violent, rattling cough with every breath, Unable to bring up any mucus, Suffocates and gags with cough, Feeling of weight on chest.	Moist, warm wind Lying down	

REMEDIES FOR EMERGENCIES

Remedy	General Indications	Worse From	Better From
For Bleeding	Bright red blood, Gushing, Gasping for air, Nosebleed, Severe nausea, Weak pulse, Cold sweat		
Ledum For Eye injury (internally and lotion)	For pain after *Arnica* fails to relieve	Night, Heat of the bed	Cold applications
Nux vomica For Asthma	Attack often follows stomach upset with much belching, Oppressed breathing with shallow respiration, Tight, dry, hacking cough, Cough brings on bursting headache, Irritable, Hypersensitive	Morning, Mental exertion, After eating, Touch Dry weather, Cold	Evening, Uninterrupted nap, Damp wet weather, Strong pressure
Phosphorus For Bleeding	Profuse bleeding anywhere, Nosebleed: profuse or from vigorous blowing	Twilight, Lying on left or painful side	Lying on right side, Dark, Cold
For Conditions with fever	Thirst for cold drinks, Appears well despite high temperature, Cold travel to chest, Cough, Sweats at night	Touch, Physical or mental exertion, Warm food or drink, Getting wet in hot weather, Ascending stairs	Cold food, Open air, Sleep, Washing in cold water

REMEDIES FOR EMERGENCIES

Remedy	General Indications	Worse From	Better From
Pulsatilla For Fainting	From hot, stuffy atmosphere	Heat, After eating	Open air, Motion Cold applications
Pyrogen For Conditions with fever	Aching, Pulse and temperature out of proportion, Restless; bed feels too hard		Motion
For Blood poisoning			
Ruta graveolens For Eye injury	Eye-strain followed by headache Painful, red, hot eyes	Lying down Cold, wet weather	Cool fresh air
Sabina For Bleeding	Uterine hemorrhage	Least motion Heat, Warm air	
Symphytum For Eye injury	Injury to eyeball, Pain in eye following a blow of blunt object		
Veratrum album For Heat exhaustion	Nausea, Pallor, Prostration, Pulse rapid and feeble, Clammy sweat, Weakness	Night, Wet, cold weather	Walking, Warmth

Actions in an Emergency

1. Assess the Situation
Are there any risks to you or the casualty?

YES

- Put your safety first
- If possible, remove the casualty
- If not possible, remove the casualty from danger when it is safe?

NO

2. Assess the Casualty
Is the casualty visibly conscious? If he has collapsed, does he respond to shaking of the shoulders?

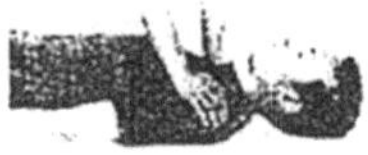

YES

- Treat the casualty and call for an ambulance, if necessary.

NO

3. Assess the Conditions
Is the condition due to injury, drowning or is the casualty a child?

YES

Are You Alone?

YES

- Move on to step 4 and carry out the resuscitation sequence **for one minute** before calling an ambulance.

NO

- Ask a helper to call an ambulance, and to pass on details of the casualty's condition.
- Move on to step 4 and carry out the resuscitation sequence.

NO

Are You Alone?

NO

- Ask a helper to call an ambulance, and to pass on details of the casualty's condition.
- Move on to step 4 and carry out the resuscitation sequence.

YES

- Move on to step 4.

Carry out resuscitation sequence. **If breathing is absent,** call an ambulance immediately.

4. Opens the Airway check breathing

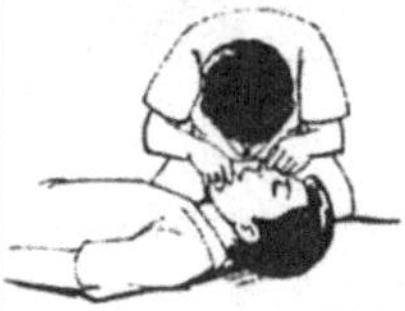

Gently tilt the casualty head well back and check for signs of breathing.
Is the casualty breathing?

YES

- Place the casualty in the recovery position .

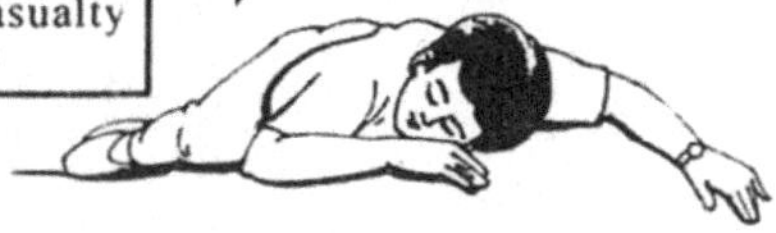

NO

5. Breathing for the casualty

Adult: Give two breaths of mouth-to-mouth ventilation.

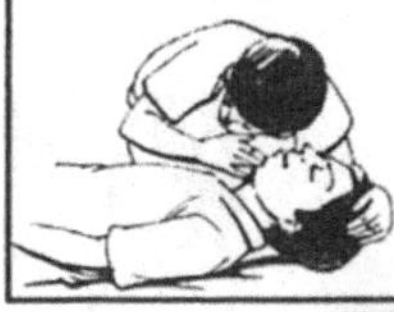

Children: Give ventilations.
Has breathing returned?

YES (to recovery position)

NO

6. Assess for circulation

Feel for a pulse for up to ten seconds and look for signs of recovery.

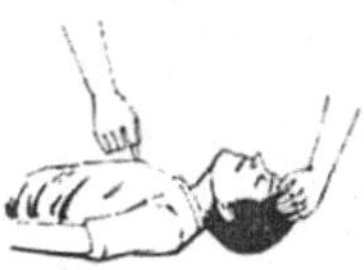

Is there a pulse or any sign of circulation?

- Continue with ventilations.
- Check the pulse and look for signs of recovery after every minute.

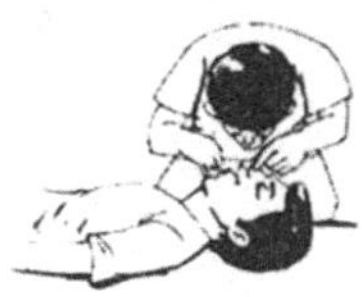

NO

7. Commence CPR

Adult: Alternate 15 chest compressions with two ventilations, repeat as needed.

Child/Baby: Give five compressions to one ventilation.

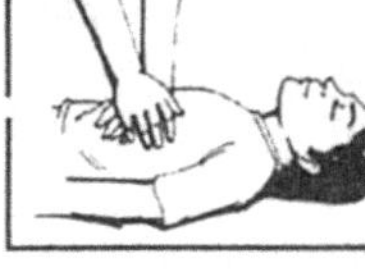

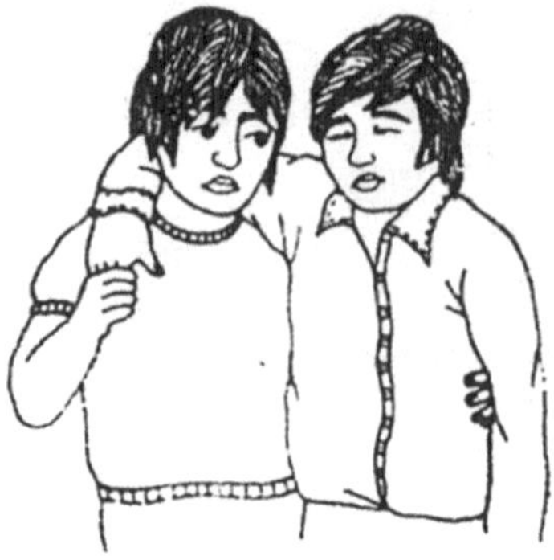

Human crutch

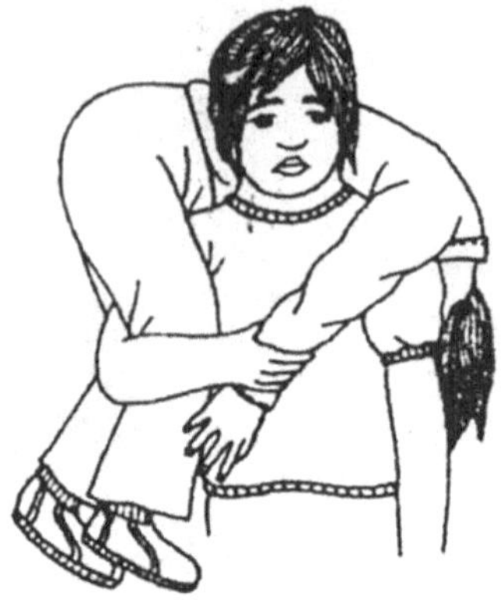

Fireman's life

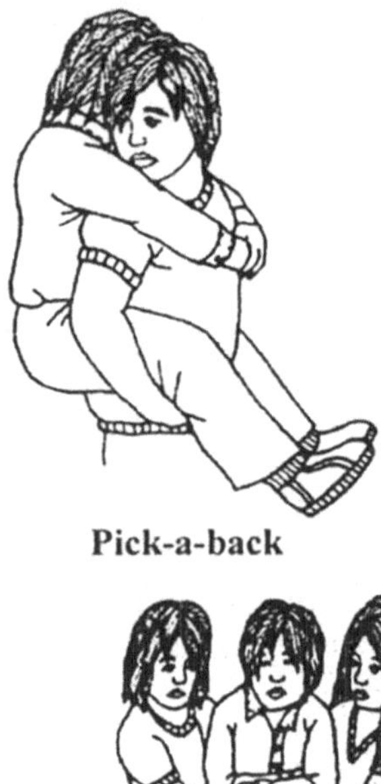

Pick-a-back

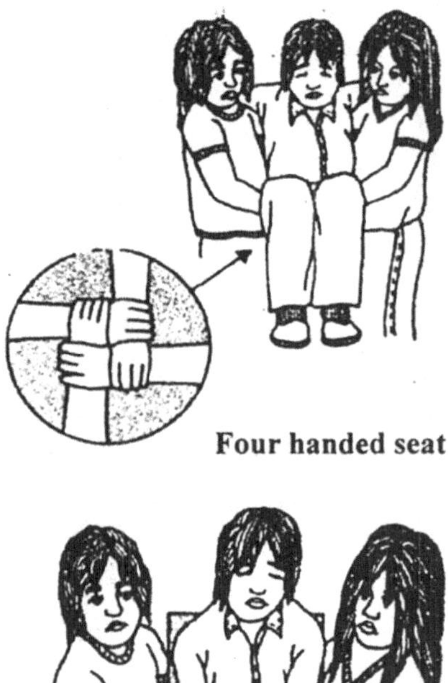

Four handed seat

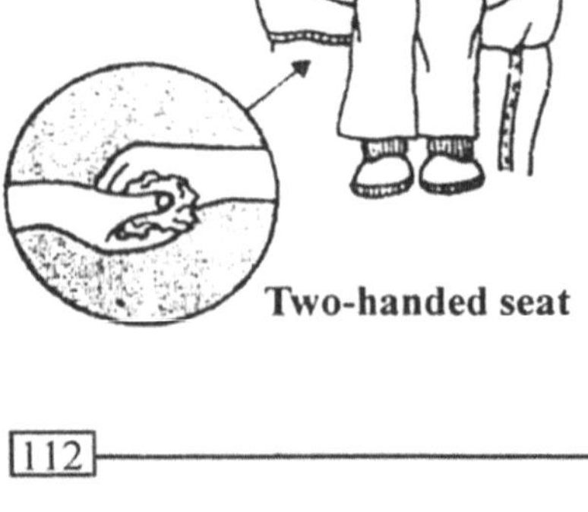

Two-handed seat

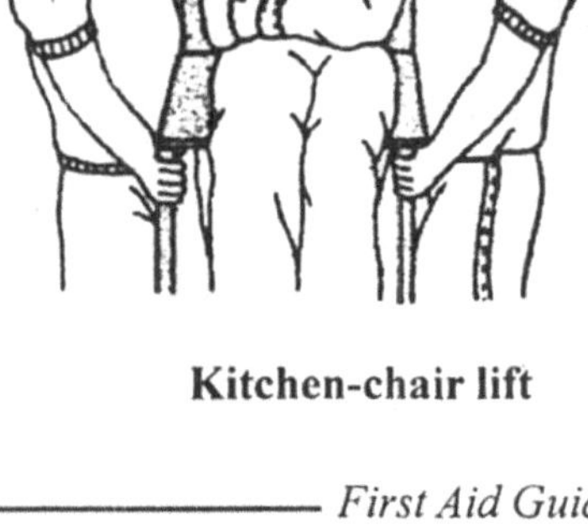

Kitchen-chair lift

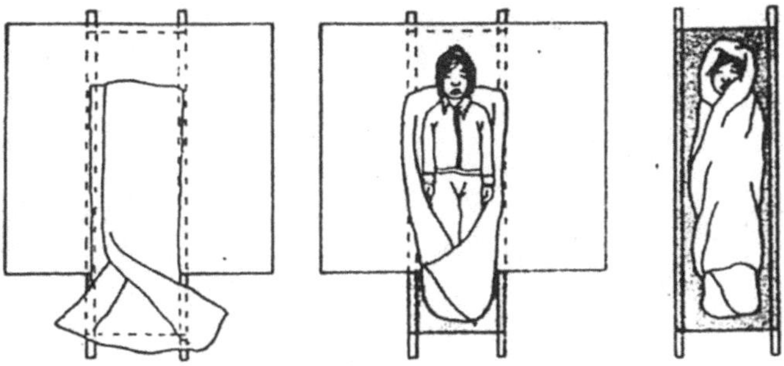

The two-blanket stretcher

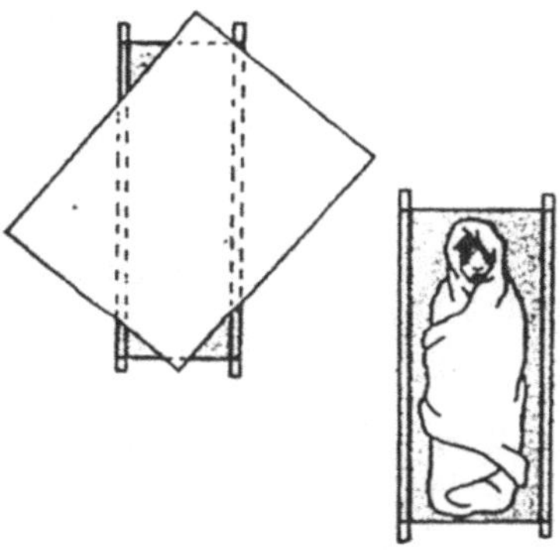

One-blanket stretcher

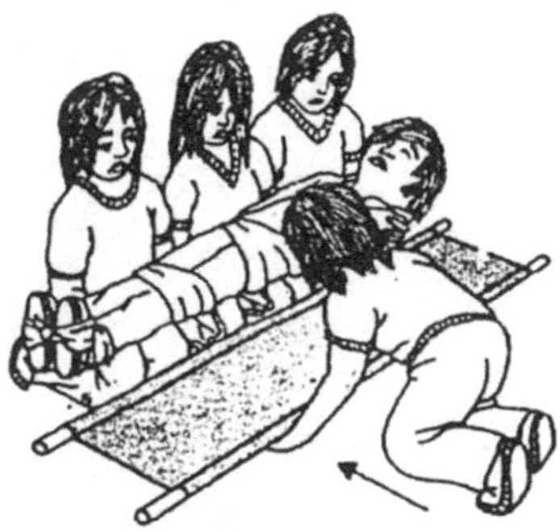

Four people load a stretcher

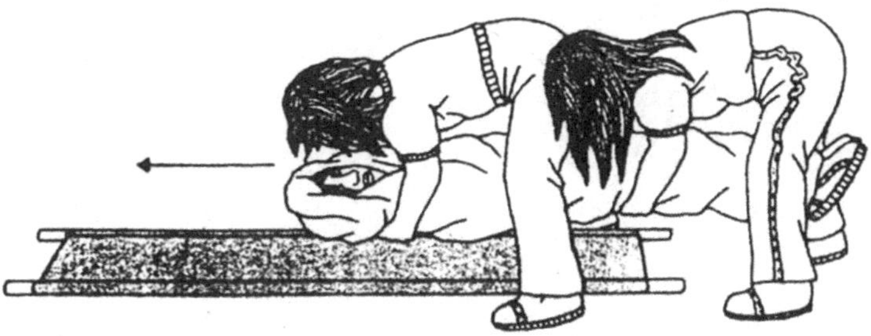

Two-bearer lift to load a stretcher

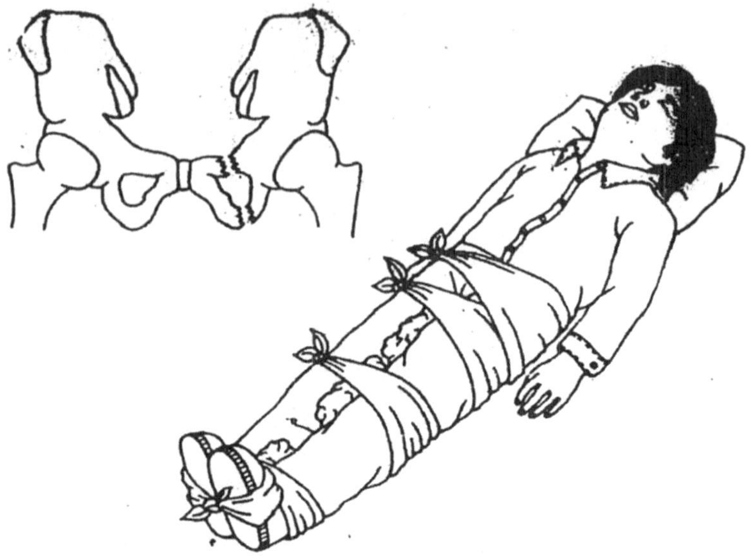

Fractured hip bone

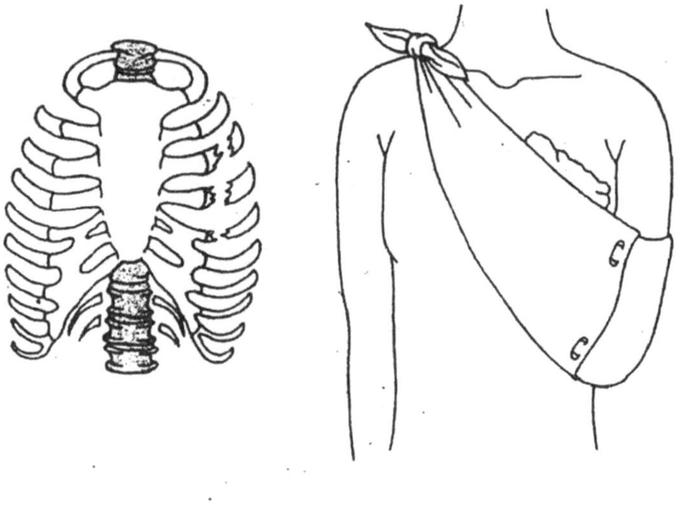

Cracked ribs

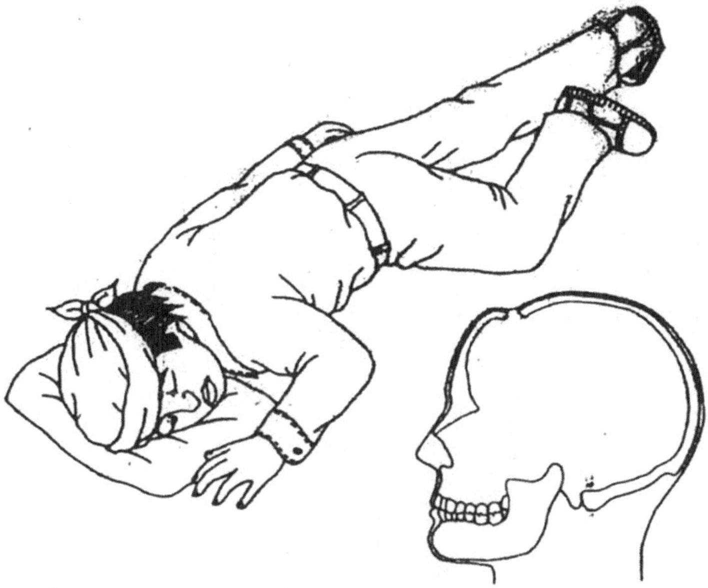

A fractured skull

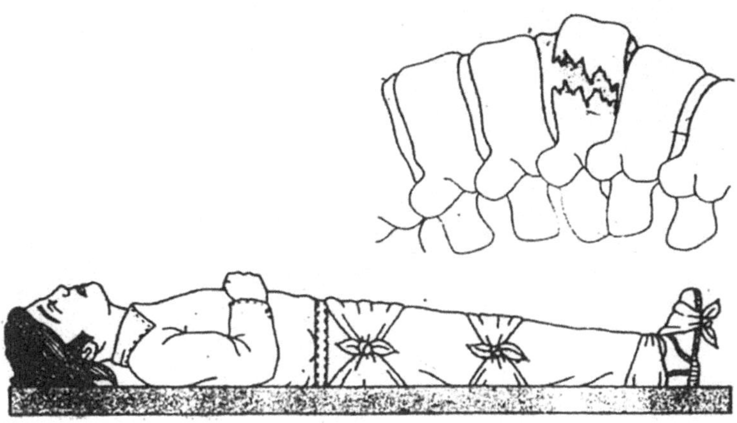

Broken spine

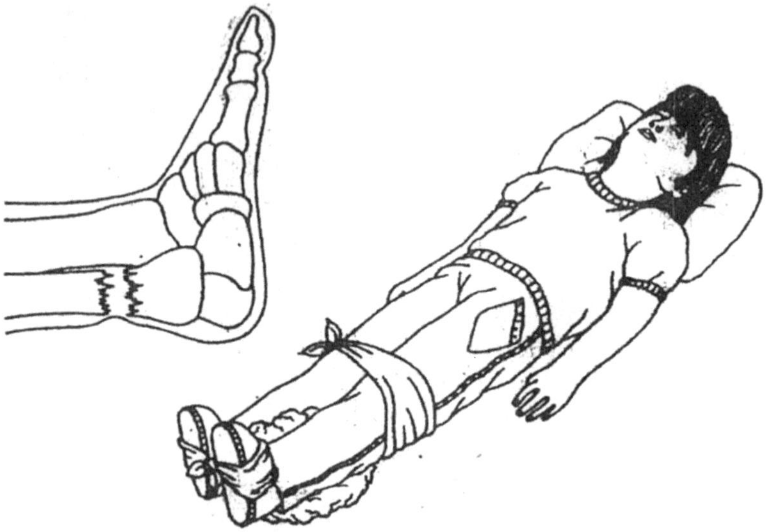

A fractured ankle

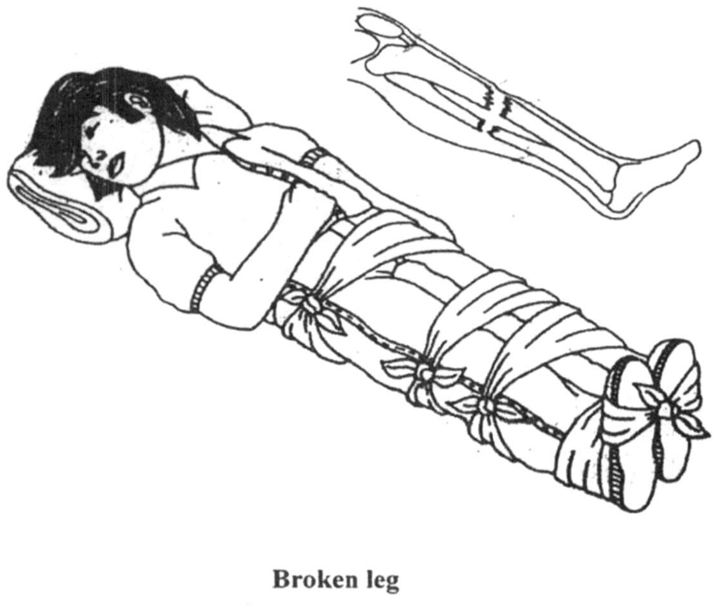

Broken leg

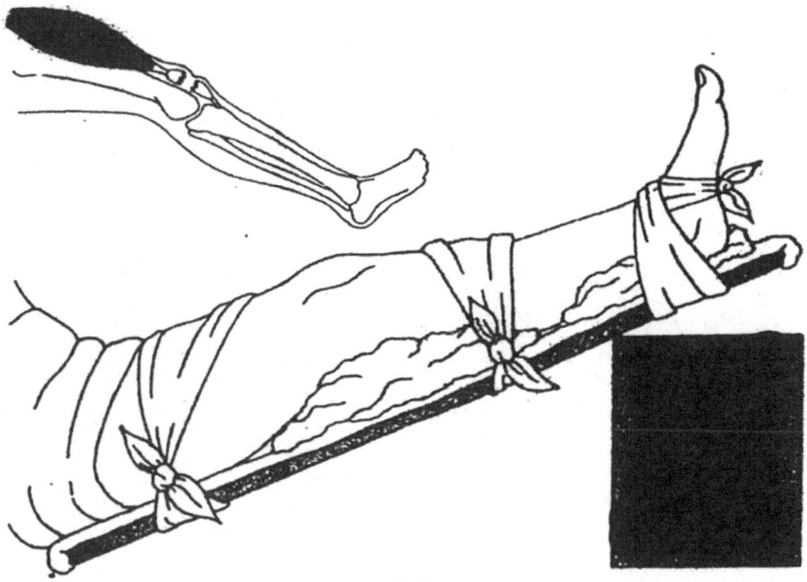

A broken knee cap

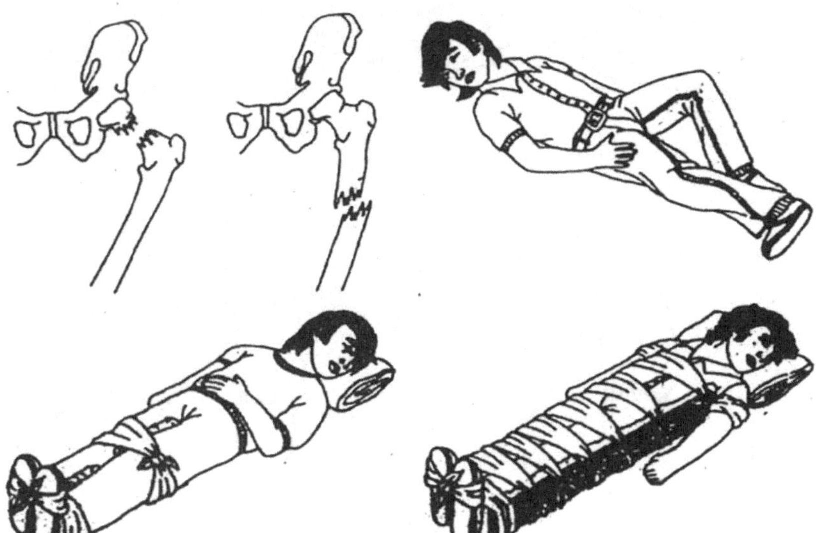

Fractured thigh bone

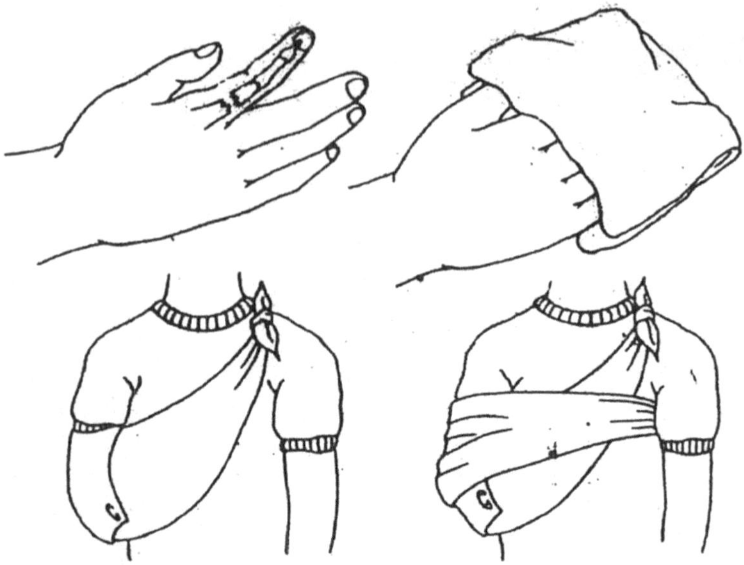

A broken finger

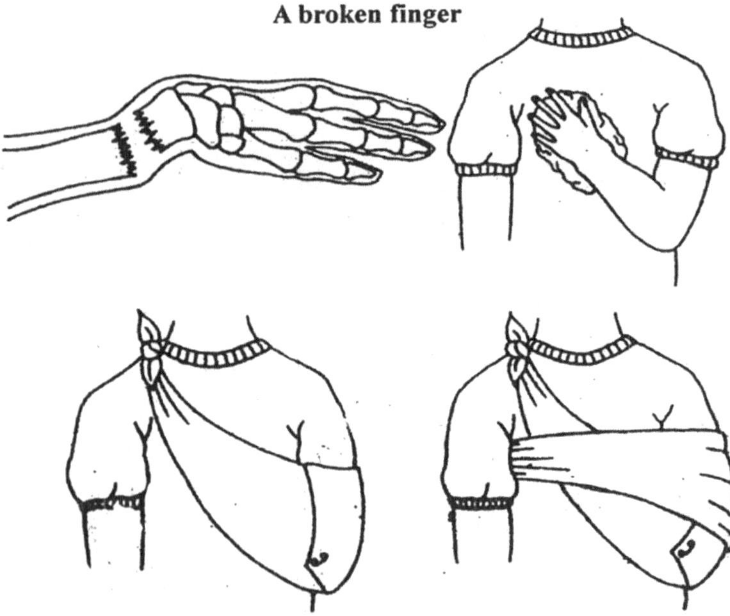

Fractured wrist

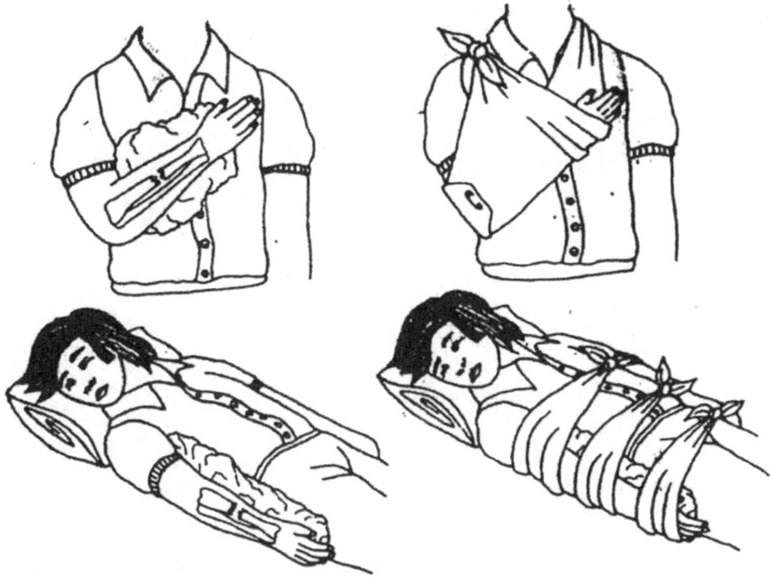

A break in the bone of arm

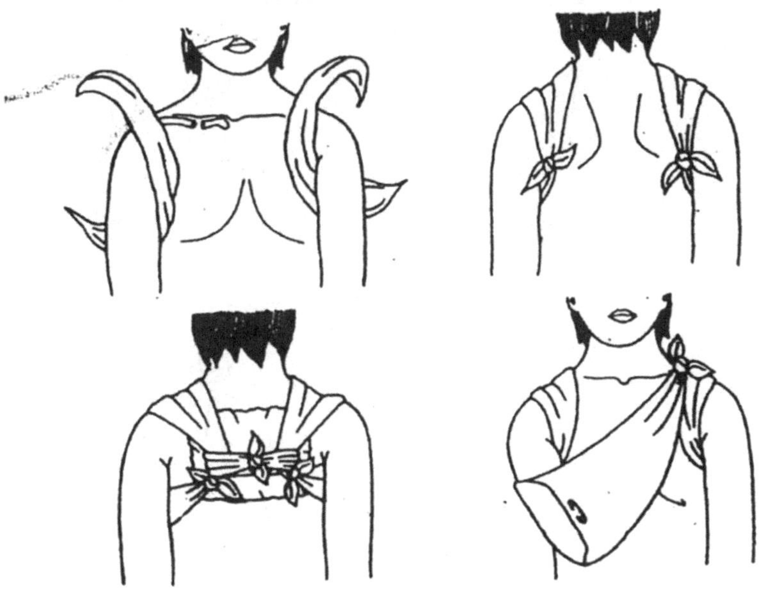

Cracked collar bone

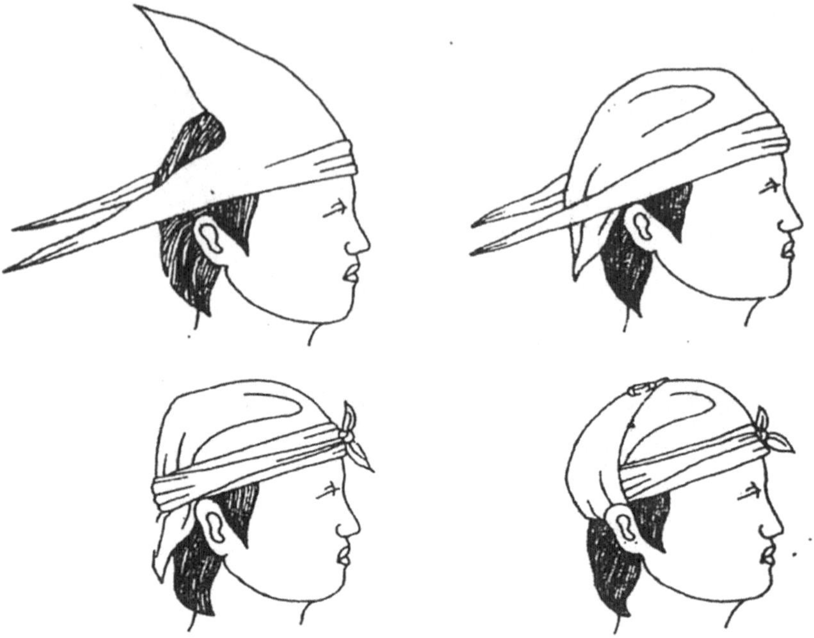

Binding the head with a triangular bandage

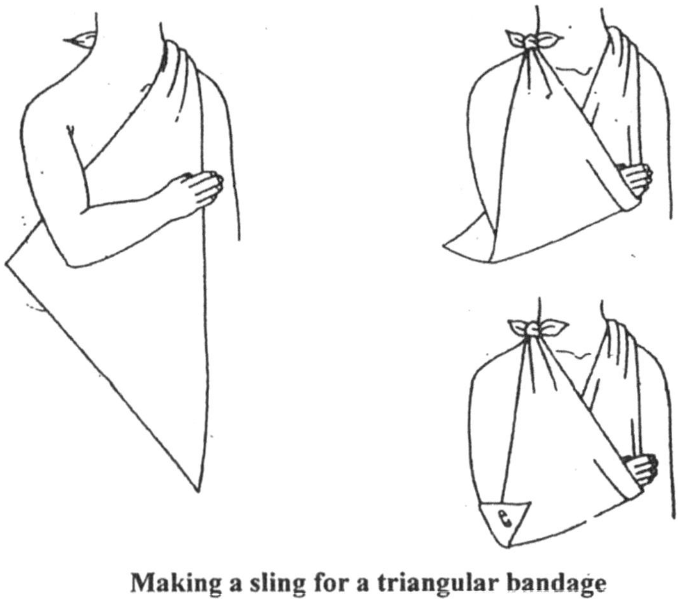

Making a sling for a triangular bandage

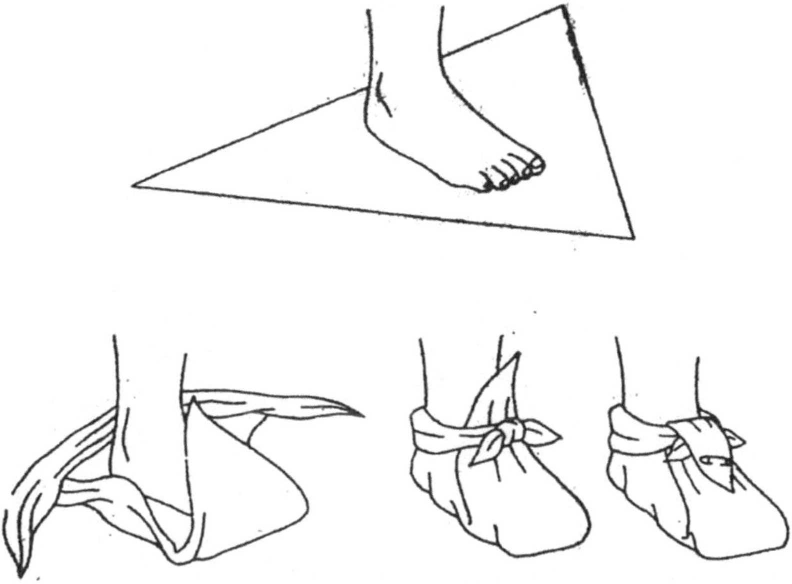

Bandaging the foot

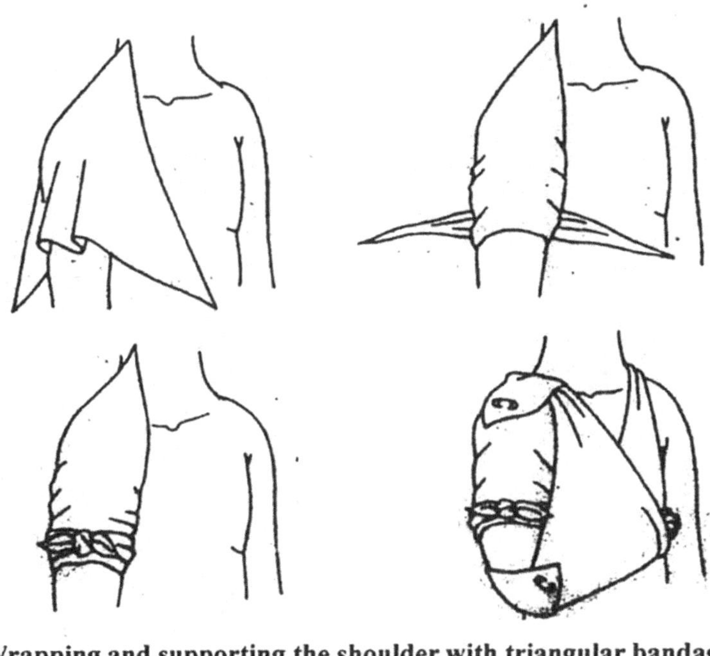

Wrapping and supporting the shoulder with triangular bandages

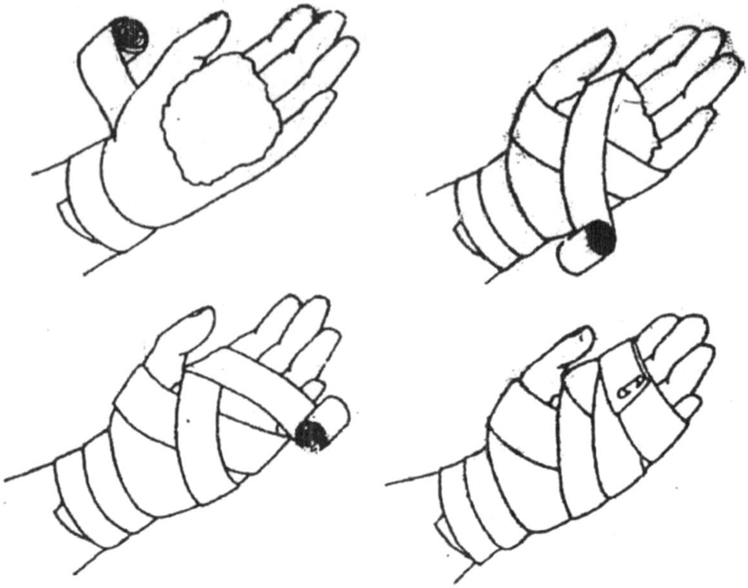

A two-inch bandage for the hand

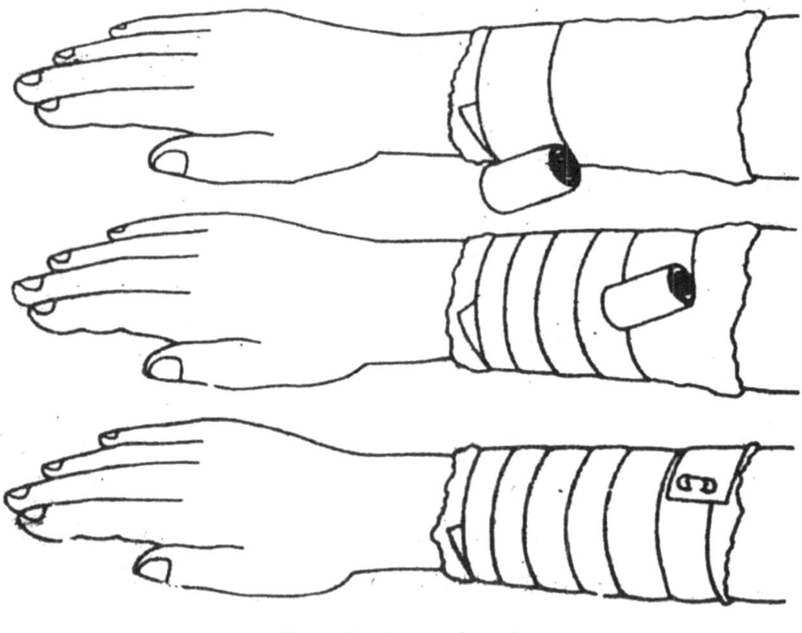

Four-inch arm bandage

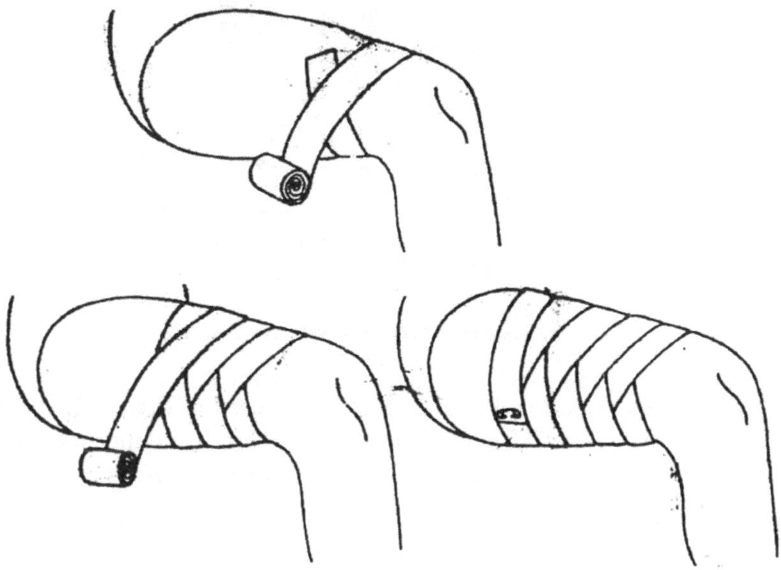

A six-inch roller bandage for the thigh

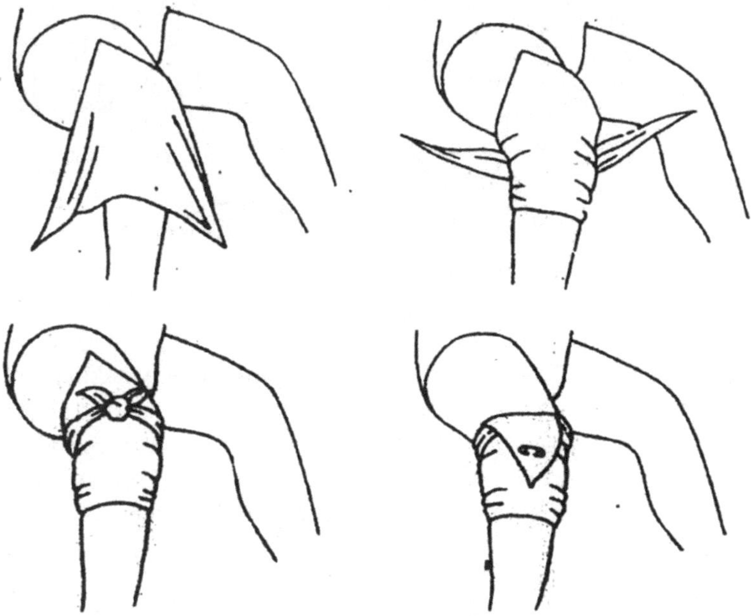

Triangular bandage around the knee

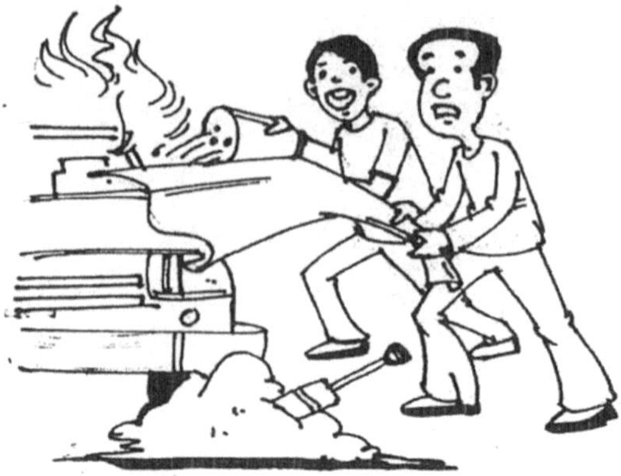

A fire extinguisher, blanket or earth may be used to fight a fire, but an explosion may occur. If there is a fire move yourself and the victim away immediately. Never use water as this may spread the flames.

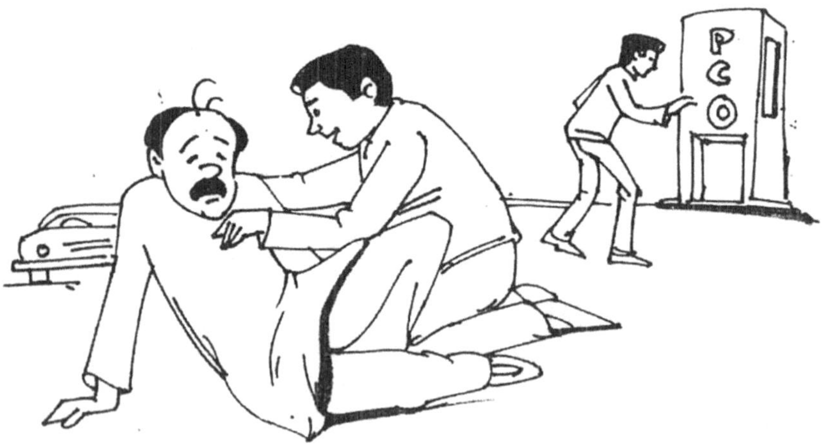

Redirect traffic: Do not rush on to the road without first making sure that it is safe to cross. Switch off the car's engine and disconnect the battery if possible. Set reflective triangles or other warning devices some 50 metres on both sides of the accident. If there is fast moving traffic on the road the warning triangles should be moved even further from the crash.

Sent for Help

Check the victim: If he is not breathing start immediate mouth-to-mouth resuscitation; if the heart has stopped initiate external cardiac compression. **Do not move the victim:** Unless the car is on fire, he is in danger of being hit by oncoming traffic, or his breathing or heart has stopped, the victim should not be disturbed.

Do not smoke: Petrol may have spilled on the roadway and the cigarette could cause a fire or explosion.

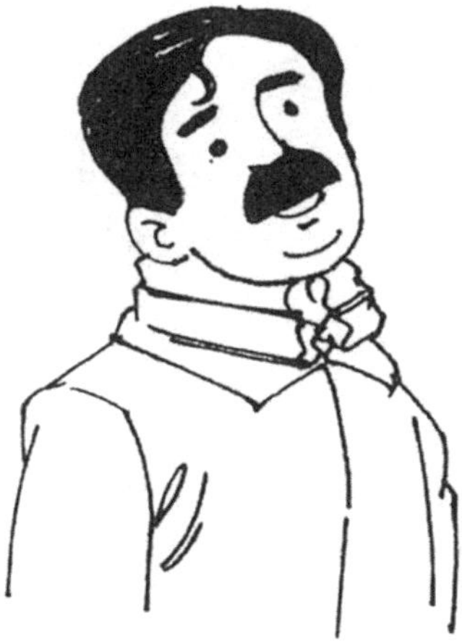

Spinal Injury

Rolling a newspaper around the neck would secure it and reduce further injury.

This chapter "Actions in an Emergency" is an illustrative guide to teach the readers, the right approach in helping the victims of casualty.

In fact the complete summary of the look is described by illustrations here

**"Help the mankind
Save humanity"**

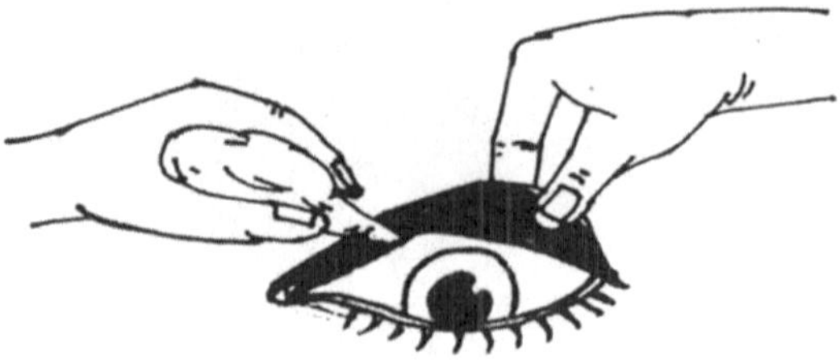

Gently wipe the foreign body in the eyes with the folded corner of a handkerchief.

Place a match stick under the eyelid and flip the lid over and over to remove the foregin body.

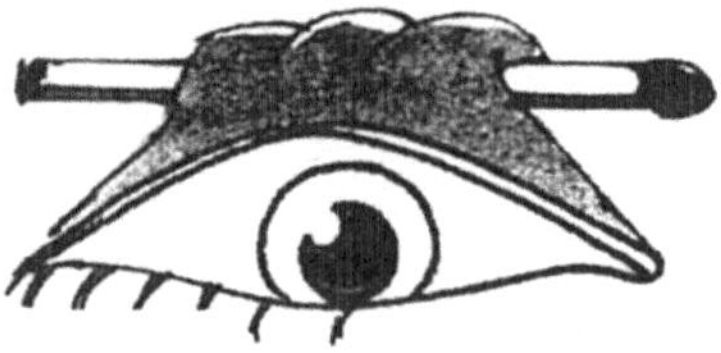

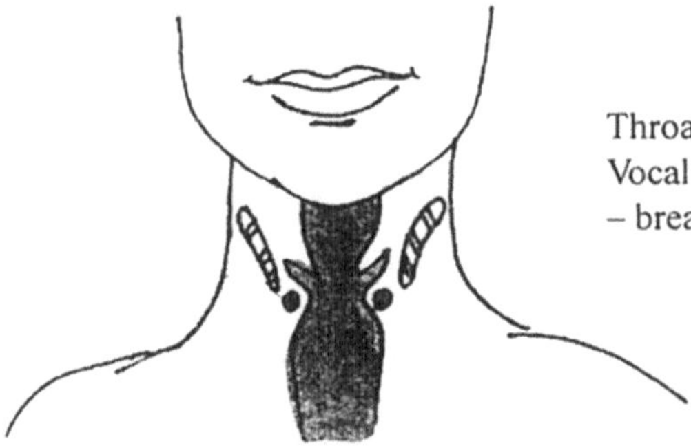

Throat clear
Vocal cord muscles relaxed
– breathing easy

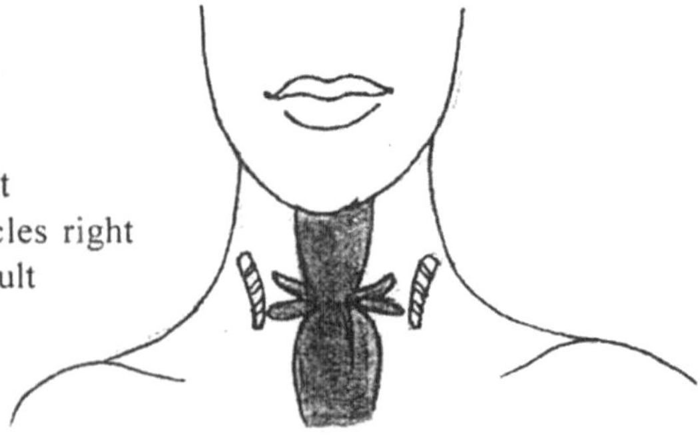

Fishbone in throat
Vocal cord muscles right
– breathing difficult

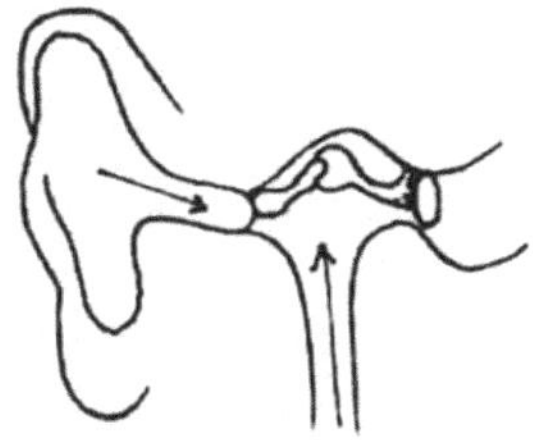

High pressure
outside ear
– blow air into
the ear.

Low Pressure
outside ear

–Swallow to
reduce the
pressure inside
the ear

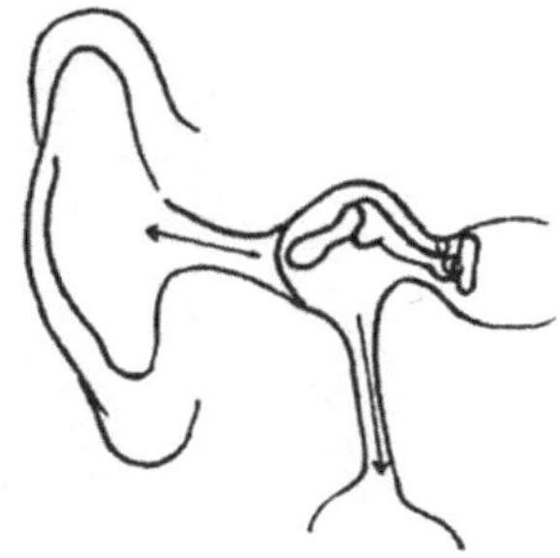

Pressure
increased caused
by inflamation
– rush to a
doctor

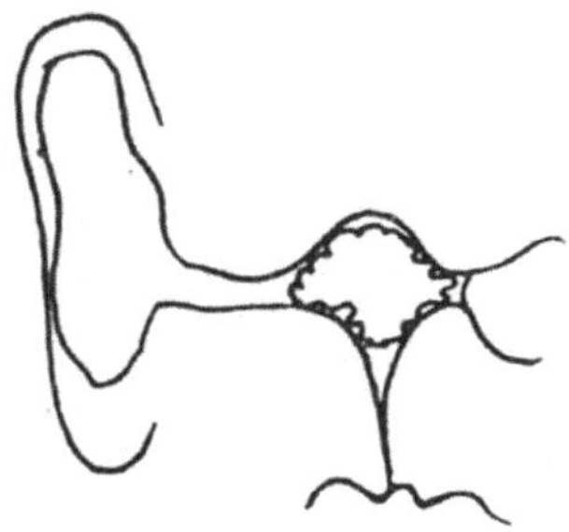

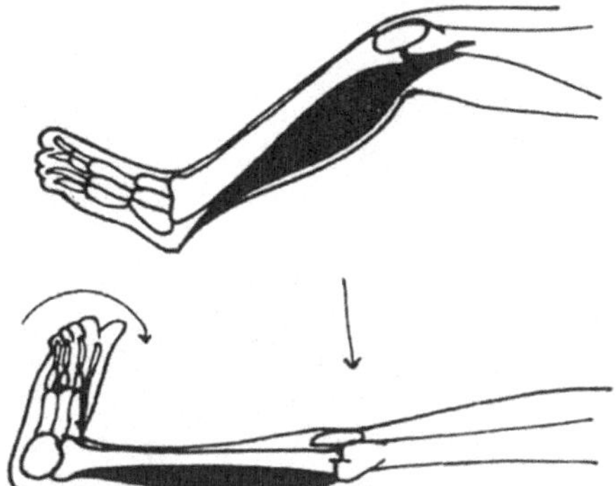

The cure for cramp is to
stretch the muscle

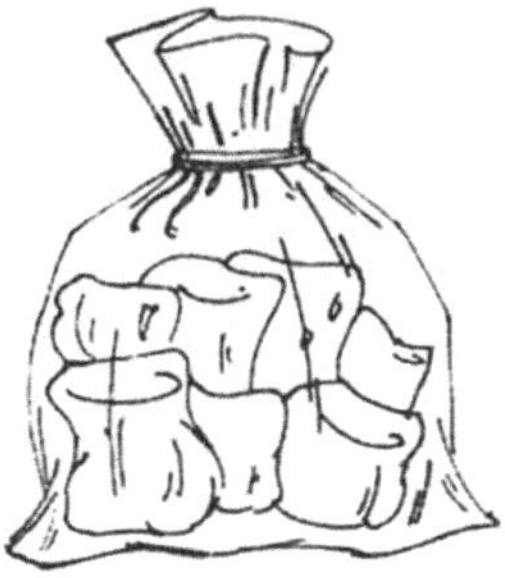

Ice pack

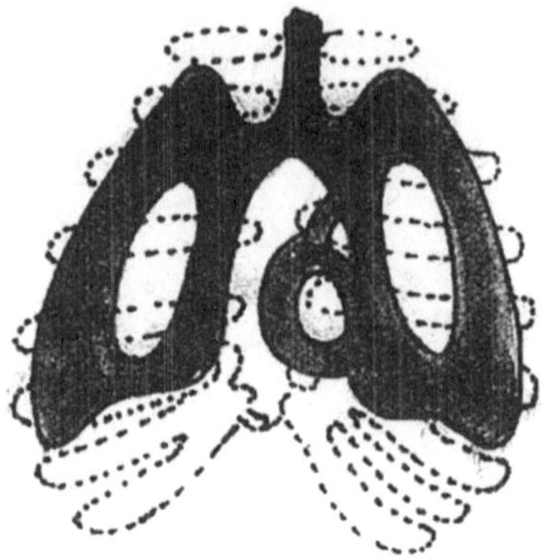

Finding the heart
A little left of centre, the heart can often be seen beating near the left nipple.

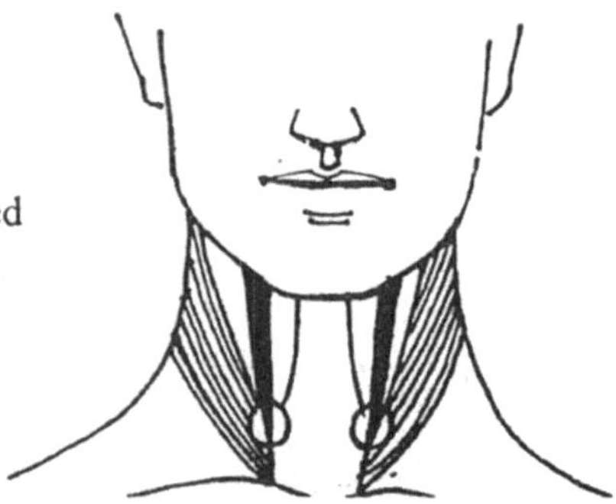

The carotid pulse
This should be checked in case of suspended cardiac arrest.

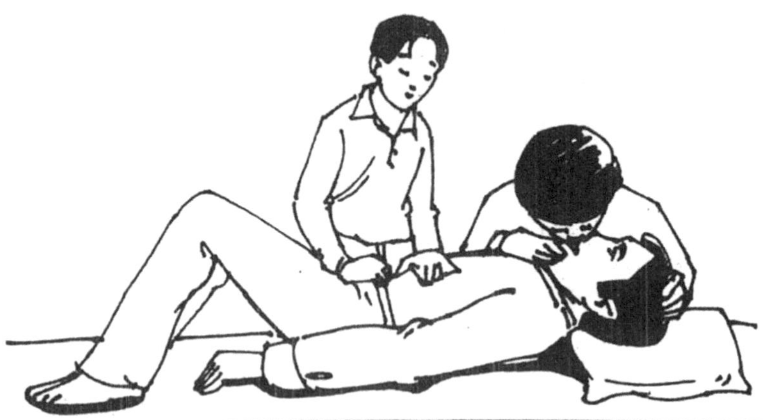

External cardiac compression with mouth-to-mouth resuscitation

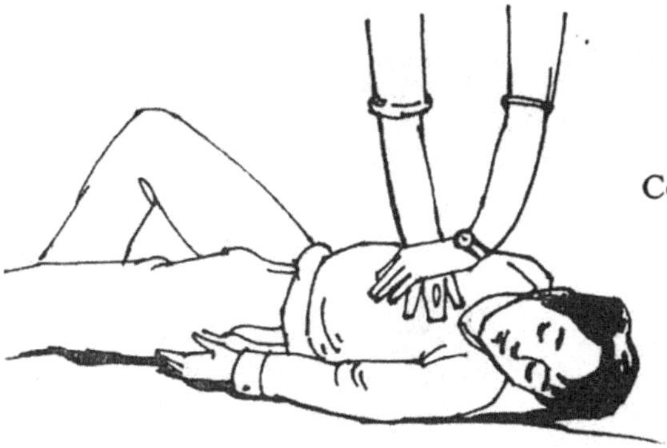

Compress the chest

Strike the lower breast bone sharply

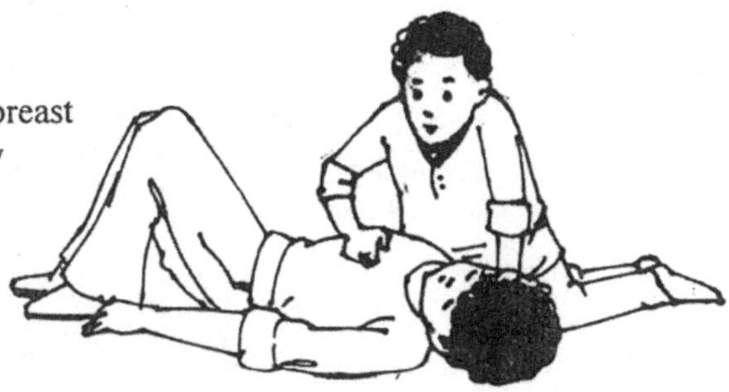

	Adult	Child	Infant
How far	5 cm.	2-4 cm.	1-2 cm.
How often	60	90	120
Where	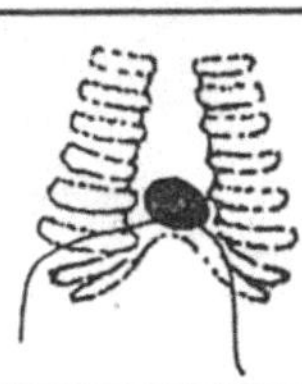	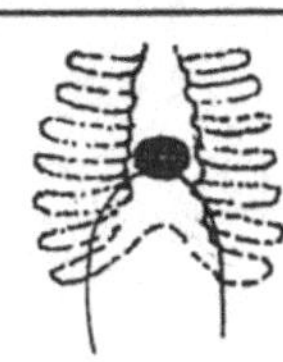	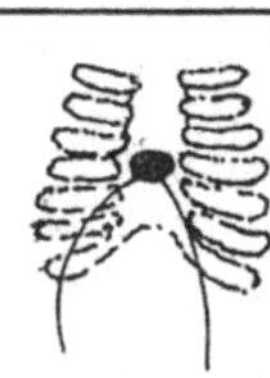
How	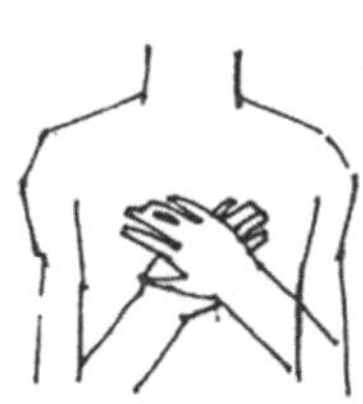	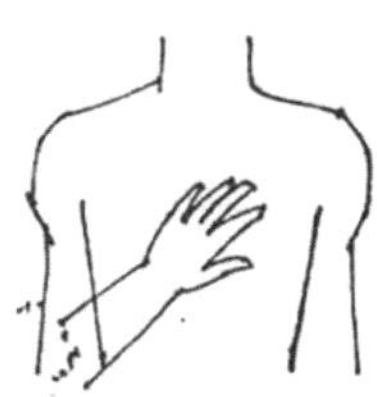	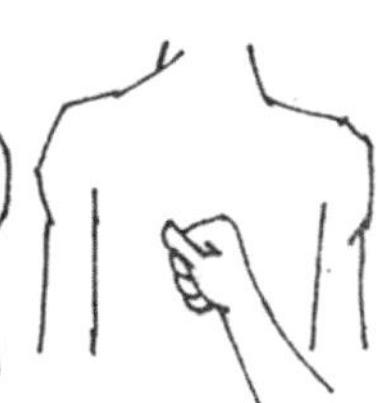

External cardiac compression in babies and young children.

Bleeding

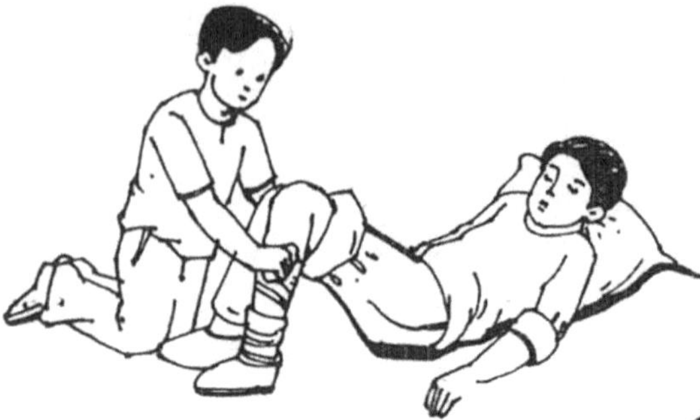

Lie the victim down and loosen the tight clothing.

Raise the wounded part.

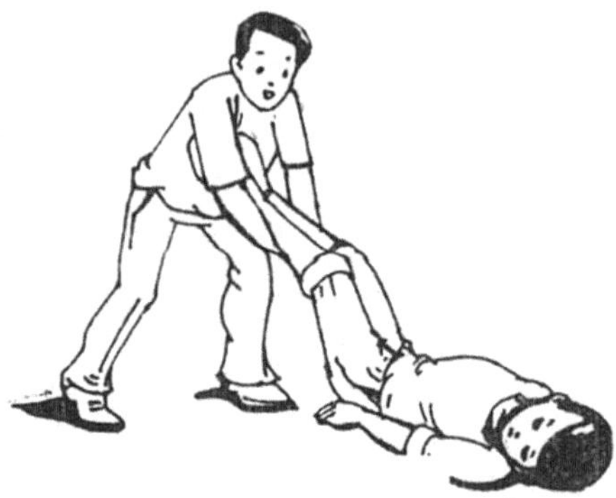

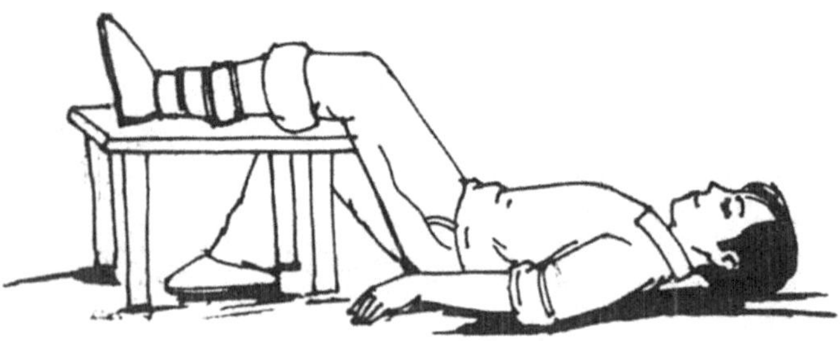

Tourniquet

Bruises

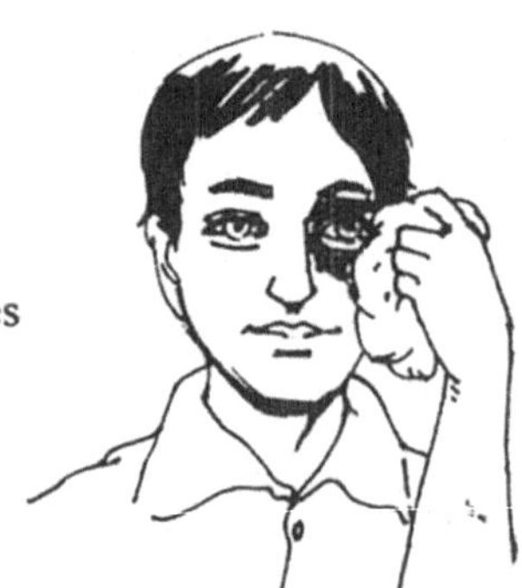

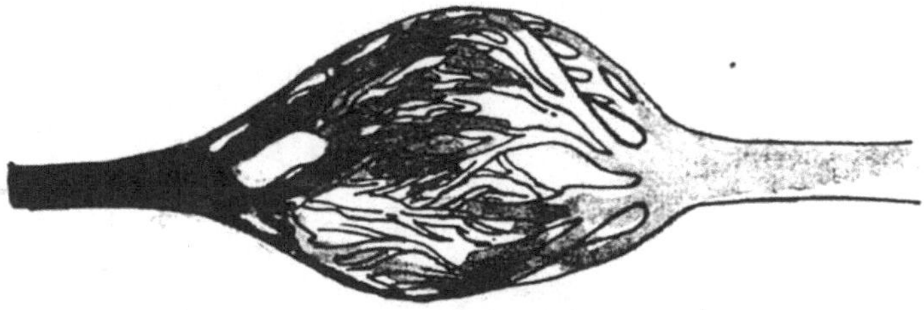

Each type of vessel bleed in a different way

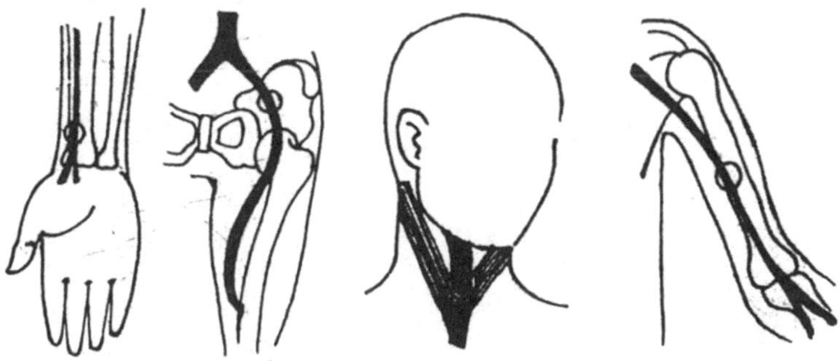

Finding the pulse and pressure points

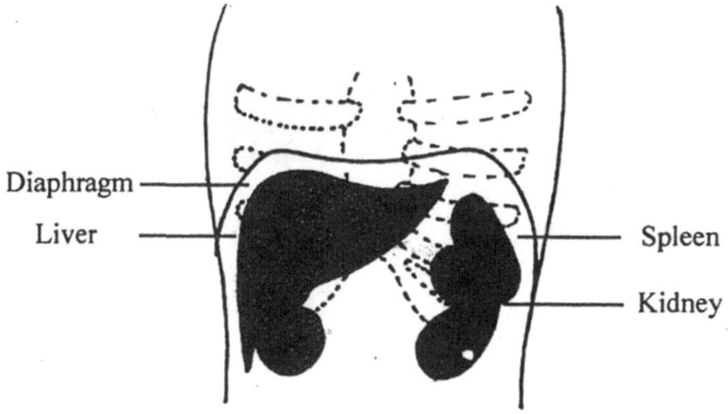

Internal Bleeding

Pulling the head back stops
the tongue blocking the airway

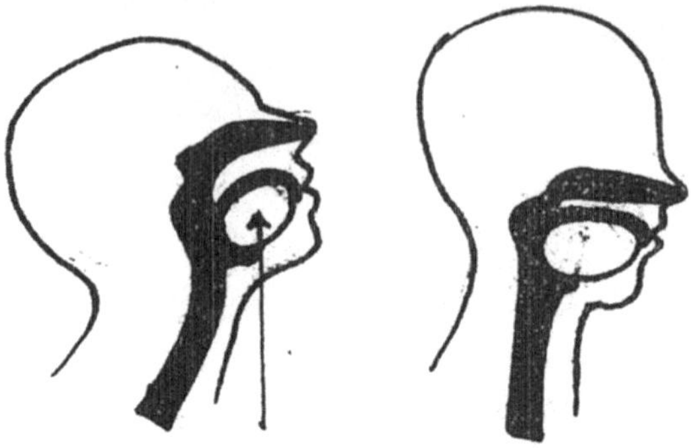

Airway open

Tongue blocks airway

When breathing stops do this

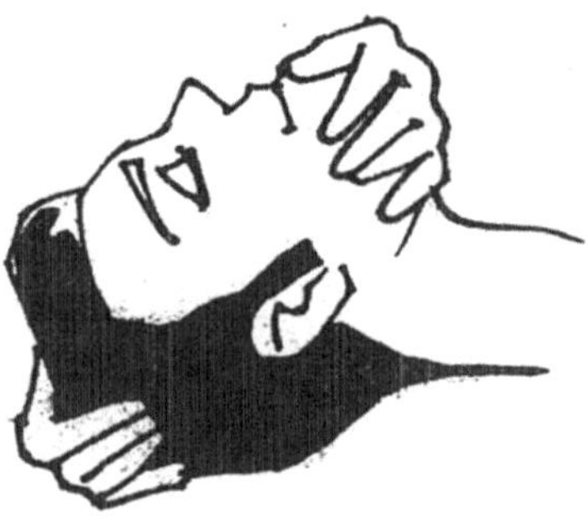

Extending the neck

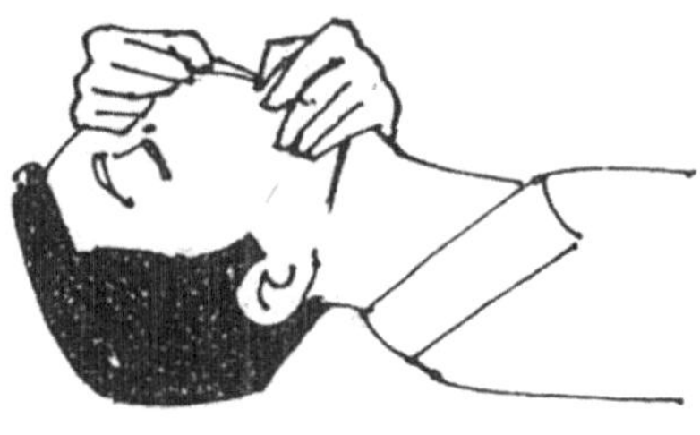

Pinching the nose and opening the mouth

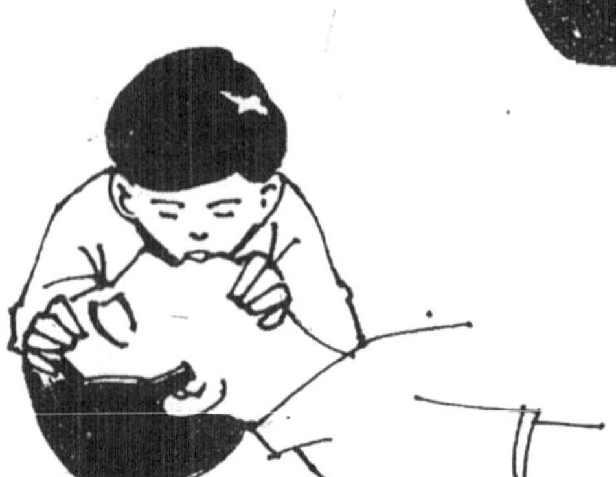

Mouth-to-mouth resuscitation

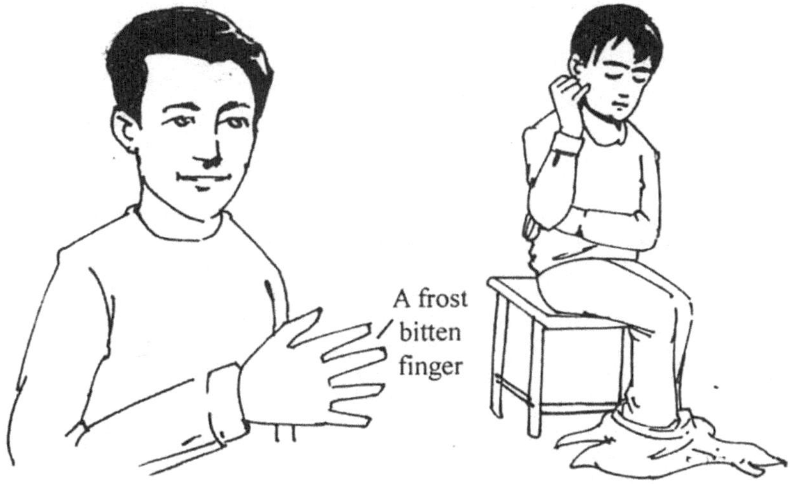

Frost bite and the first aid treatment

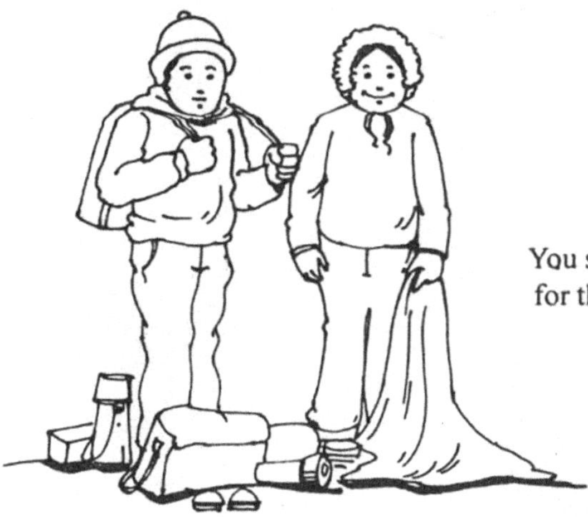

You should be prepared for the exhaustive cold

The right way to treat cold exhaustion

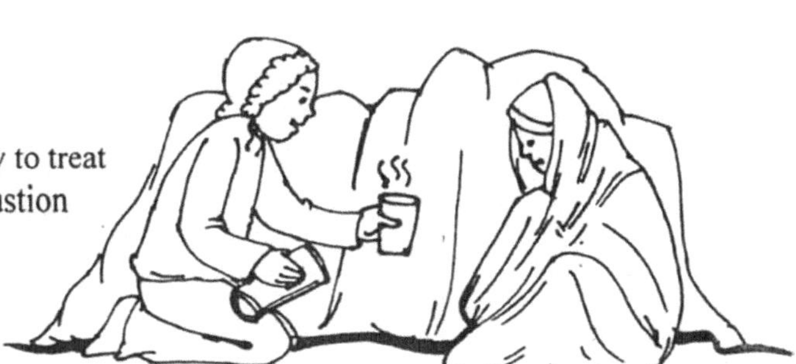

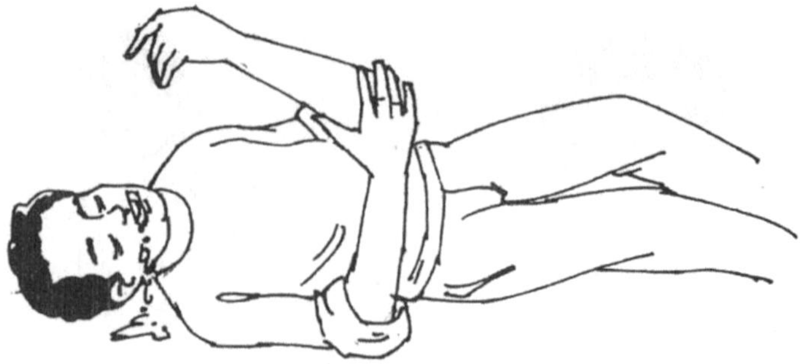

Epileptic fit

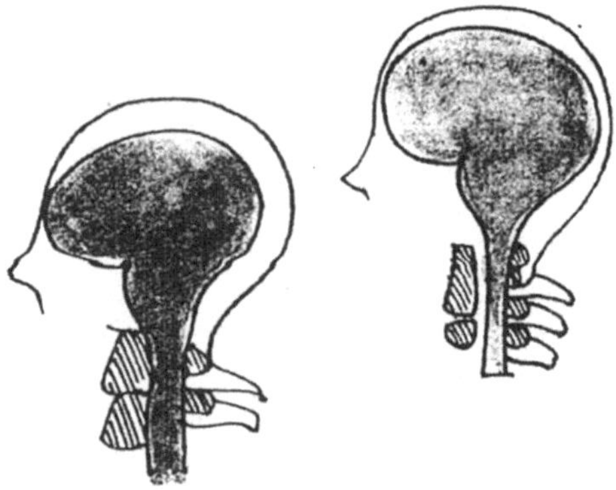

Brain concussion
(shaking)

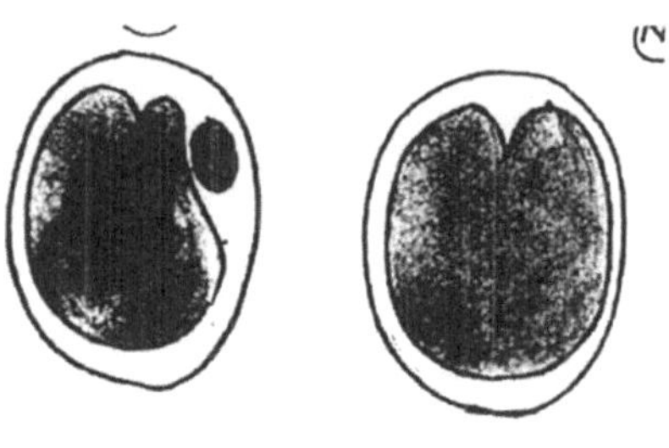

Brain compression
(bleeding)

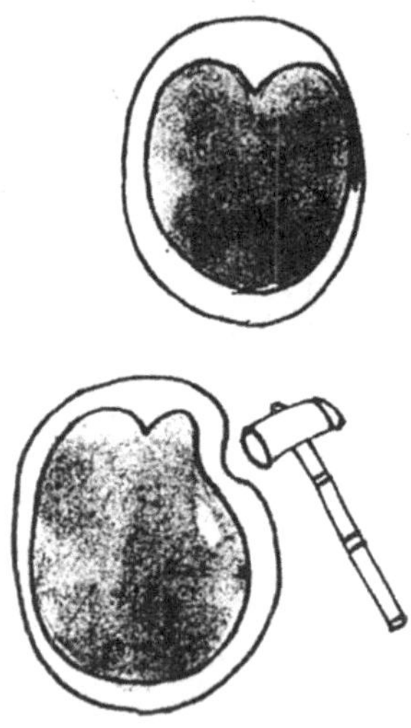

Brain compression
(fracture)

BOOKS ON SELF-HELP

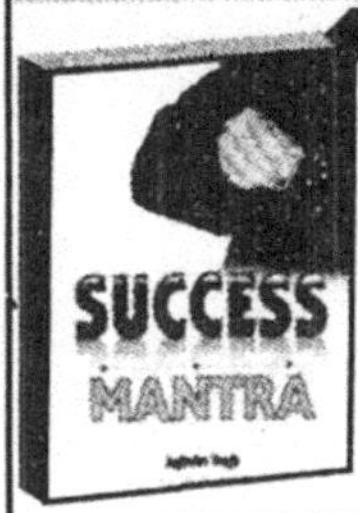

Rs 150/-

SUCCESS MANTRA (Sh. Joginder Singh)

This book is a masterpiece by Sh. Joginder Singh, IPS (Retd) who is a former Director of the CBI. Hailing from a poor farmer's family, he scaled the pinnacles of success through sheer motivation and hard work. The saga of success he has enunciated through his win-win story is worth emulating for any young aspirant for achievements and glory in life: to be on top!

HOW TO EXCEL WHEN CHIPS ARE DOWN

Rs 95/-

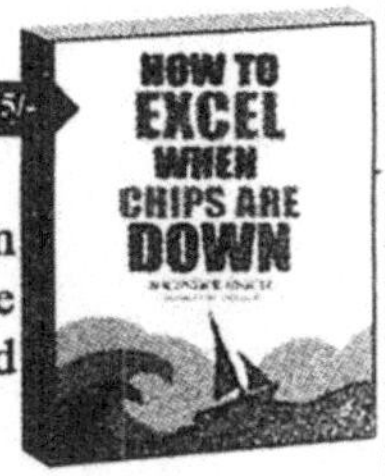

(Sh. Joginder Singh)

Excellent suggestions with suitable examples have been cited in the book which will guide youngesters about the importance of objective thinking and to erase unwanted thoughts from their memory.

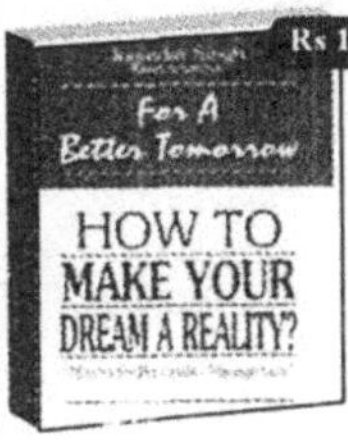

Rs 150/-

FOR A BETTER TOMORROW (Sh. Joginder Singh)

This magnum opus by Sh. Joginder Singh is a treatise on self improvement. This win-win sory is based on the secrets of success as to how to become an achiever. And the success mantra that he espouses for you. Make the best of all opportunities; 'dream big and work hard- dreams will turn sheer realities.

WINNING WAYS

Rs 150/-

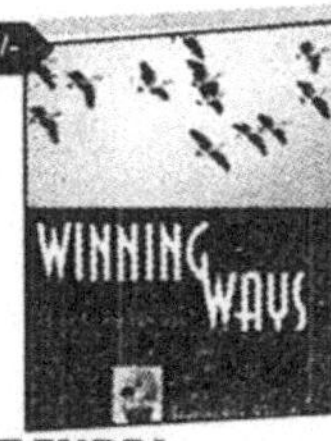

(Sh. Joginder Singh)

The mantra he unveils for success, through this book, is potent enough to lift the young and ambitious to the highest peaks. These winning tips will inspire your morale to achieve greater glories - you simply need to tune up your mindset and hone your skills.

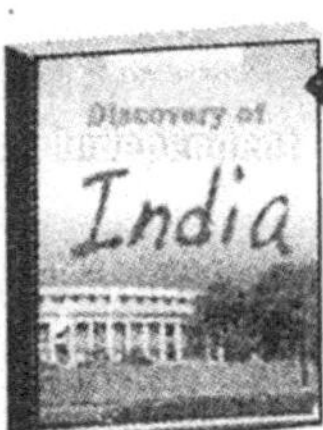

Rs 95/-

DISCOVERY OF INDEPENDENT INDIA

By: Joginder Singh (Former CBI Director)

Violation of human rights does not occur only at the hands of the enforcement agencies. Rampant corruption in Govt. department will whom a citizen comes across at the cutting edge level, tell their own story. The biggest hurdle which inhibits the citizen from coming forward to help the police is the deplorable condition prevailing in the Court of law.

TURN YOUR CREATIVE SPARK INTO A FLAME

Joginder Singh

Rs 95/-

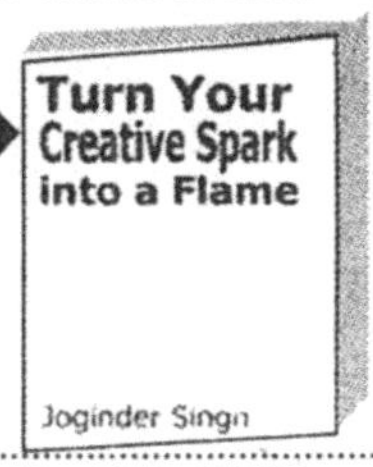

This book explains the significance of motivating today's youngesters and other aspirants on various aspects. It acts as an eye-opener about the common mistakes that everyone commit in their lives, that is badly managing the schedules and wastage of the precious time of our life.

DIAMOND BOOKS

X-30, Okhla Industrial Area, Phase-II, New Delhi-110020,
Phones : 41611861- 65, 40712100, Fax: 011- 41611866
E-mail : Sales@dpb.in, Website: www.dpb.in